# Medical-Surgical Nursing Care Plans

## Nursing Diagnosis and Interventions

**Linda Skidmore-Roth, R.N., M.S.N.**
Formerly Nursing Faculty
New Mexico, State University
Las Cruces, New Mexico

Formerly Nursing Faculty
El Paso Community College
El Paso, Texas

**Marie Jaffe, R.N., M.S.**
Formerly Nursing Faculty
University of Texas at El Paso
El Paso, Texas

 **APPLETON-CENTURY-CROFTS/Norwalk, Connecticut**

0-8385-6279-5

Copyright © 1986 by Appleton-Century-Crofts
A Publishing Division of Prentice-Hall

86  87  88  89  90  /  10  9  8  7  6  5  4  3  2  1

Prentice-Hall of Australia, Pty. Ltd., Sydney
Prentice-Hall Canada, Inc.
Prentice-Hall Hispanoamericana, S.A., Mexico
Prentice-Hall of India Private Limited, New Delhi
Prentice-Hall International (UK) Limited, London
Prentice-Hall of Japan, Inc., Tokyo
Prentice-Hall of Southeast Asia (Pte.) Ltd., Singapore
Whitehall Books Ltd., Wellington, New Zealand
Editora Prentice-Hall do Brasil Ltda., Rio de Janeiro

**Library of Congress Cataloging-in-Publication Data**
Skidmore-Roth, Linda.
  Medical-surgical nursing care plans.

  Bibliography: p.
  Includes index.
  1. Nursing care plans—Handbooks, manuals, etc.
2. Surgical nursing—Handbooks, manuals, etc.
I. Jaffe, Marie S. II. Title. [DNLM: 1. Nursing—
handbooks. 2. Patient Care Planning—handbooks.
3. Surgical Nursing—handbooks. WY 39 S628m]
RT49.S56   1986      610.73      86-10721
ISBN 0-8385-6279-5

Design: Jean Sabato-Morley
Cover: M. Chandler Martylewski

# Contents

# Preface

Developing individualized nursing care plans is necessary for providing optimum patient care in a variety of health care settings. This book was written as a reference for the improvement of nursing care plans in the clinical area. It is to be used by nursing students, practicing nurses, and quality assurance coordinators in medical-surgical areas of hospitals, outpatient clinics, physician offices and staff development departments.

This text is the distillation of many years as both educators and practitioners in various medical-surgical areas in hospitals and outpatient clinics. During the years in these areas, we noticed the difficulty both beginning as well as advanced students, and practicing nurses, have in generation of individualized nursing care plans. Many books are now on the market that contain general nursing care plans. However, there is need for specific plans that include assessment guides for each system, nursing diagnoses that conform to those defined by the North American Nursing Diagnosis Association, goals that provide outcome criteria, and interventions with rationales.

Our purpose for this text is twofold: first, to provide a conceptual base for nursing care planning; second, to provide a quick reference for all nurses who are responsible for planning patient care. These plans are standards for practice in the medical-surgical area.

We wish to express our gratitude to our families and friends who provided emotional support during the writing of the text. Appreciation is also expressed to Pam Garrard for the efficient typing of the manuscript. Finally, we are grateful for the support and encouragement of Rick Weimer and Marion Kalstein-Welch.

Linda Skidmore-Roth
Marie Jaffe

# How to Use This Book

This book was designed and developed for use in medical-surgical settings as a quick reference. It is not intended to be used as a primary text; rather, it is an informational resource for those responsible for the management of the patient care in medical-surgical conditions. Nursing students as well as new and experienced staff nurses in these units will benefit from the content and it is hoped that their use of this book will result in more efficient and effective practices in the assessment, planning, implementation, and evaluation of nursing care.

The book is presented by systems and categories. Medical-surgical conditions, assessments and procedures are cross-indexed for easy access.

Seven divisions of information are included as follows:

**TITLE:** Identifies the condition, assessment, or procedure

**DEFINITION:** Presents a brief definition of the condition, assessment or procedure, and signs and symptoms of each condition when applicable

**CONCEPT/NEED:** Identifies the concept and/or need of possible problem area according to priority and to provide a guideline for data collection. As many concepts and/or needs are developed as necessary

**NURSING DIAGNOSIS:** Provides one example for each problem identified, which is related to the concept/need. Diagnoses conform to the North American Nursing Diagnosis Association. However, nursing diagnosis are formulated without the necessary data base and should be supplemented or changed according to individual patient needs

**GOALS:** Provides examples of goals related to the diagnoses. In all instances, the examples include the necessary criteria for expected outcomes

**INTERVENTIONS:** Lists interventions according to categories of the following:

**I. Monitor, describe, record:** This section includes areas in which astute observation is necessary

**II. Assess for:** This section includes areas in which continued assessment is needed during the patient stay

**III. Administer:** This section includes all medications and procedures needed to assist in the patient recovery. All medications are designated with "as ordered" to assist the beginning nurses in defining the dependent nursing functions

**IV. Perform/Provide:** This section includes all nursing treatments and physical therapy regimens when applicable

**V. Teach patient/family:** Includes all teaching aspects for hospitalization as well as those needed for discharge. The term "patient" is used throughout the text since most conditions included would be seen in the acute care hospital rather than in the home

The designated Roman numeral for each category is used consistently as applicable to the interventions; numerals may be skipped if there is no pertinent information in that category.

**RATIONALE:** A brief statement of a principle or reason as to why the intervention is being considered and carried out

# GENERAL STANDARDS

- ■ Health History
- ■ Safety Assessment
- ■ Diagnostic Procedures
- ■ Laboratory Tests/Specimen Collection
- ■ Pre-Operative Care
- ■ Post-Operative Care
- ■ Discharge Planning

# ■ Health History

**DEFINITION:** The collection of data on admission by interview or investigation. This data base is used in conjunction with the physical examination, psychosocial assessment, diagnostic and laboratory test results, prescribed medications and treatments in the formulation of nursing diagnoses

## I. Identifying information:
   A. Age, sex, race, ethnicity, occupation, marital status, religion, health insurance, residence
   B. Source of information

## II. Present history:
   A. Chief complaint, patient's words if possible
   B. Onset and development of problems, where took place, what was done
   C. Signs and symptoms, their location, severity, duration, frequency, changes, effect on patient, meaning of disease to patient
   D. What alleviated or aggravated symptoms
   E. Knowledge of disease, procedures, and planned therapy
   F. Laboratory and diagnostic tests done since admission
   G. Medications and treatments given since admission

## III. Past history:
   A. Statement about general health
   B. Other medical conditions and date of onset or occurrence
   C. Previous surgeries, injuries, and dates
   D. Hospitalizations for injuries, medical problems
   E. Allergies to food, medicines, environment
   F. Immunizations and dates
   G. Military history, travel and dates
   H. Childhood diseases and ages occurred
   I. Psychiatric illness and treatment
   J. Usual health care patterns and kind of practitioner used
   K. Medications and treatments used including prescriptions, OTC, folk therapies, heating pad, and others
   L. Life style patterns and personal habits in sleep, nutrition, fluid intake, urinary and bowel elimination, activity, sexual behavior, personal hygiene, etc.

## IV. Psychosocial history:
A. Use of coffee, alcohol, tobacco, other drugs, amount, frequency, and type
B. Statement about general appearance
C. Living arrangement, significant persons and relationship
D. Occupation and income, ability to pay for health care
E. Housing, neighborhood, and feelings
F. Distance and transportation to health care
G. Education, years completed
H. Recreation and interests
I. Friends, community involvement, church attendance
J. English as a second language or no English spoken

## V. Family history:
A. Health status of parents, spouse, siblings, children, including deaths with age and cause
B. Health status of grandparents, blood relatives
C. Role and responsibilities of family members and if working outside home
D. Relationship with family members, activities, response to stress or crisis, abuse
E. Marital relationship
F. History of heart conditions, diabetes, cancer, or other diseases of family members

## VI. Review of systems:
A. Height, weight, vital signs
B. Integumentary to include rash, pruritis, lesions, dandruff, changes in color, nails, or hair
C. Neurological to include headaches, injuries, fainting, seizures, tremors, numbness, tingling, dizziness, paralysis, changes in memory, touch, taste, smell, hearing, vision, infection, pain in eyes, discharge, infection, pain, ringing in ears
D. Use of glasses, contacts, or hearing aid
E. Respiratory to include cough and characteristics, sputum, dyspnea, wheezing, hemoptysis, congestion or discharge from nose, pain in throat, nose, chest, epistaxis, throat infections, asthma, bronchitis, pneumonia, emphysema, URIs
F. Cardiovascular to include chest pain, edema, dyspnea, palpitations, hypertension, blocks, MI, phlebitis, trouble with circulation to extremities
G. Gastrointestinal to include abdominal pain, nausea, vomiting,

diarrhea, constipation, hemorrhoids, indigestion, swallowing, appetite, excessive flatus, or belching, changes in stool color, consistency, or frequency, mouth, teeth, or chewing problems, hepatitis, diverticulitis, gallstones, peptic ulcer, colitis, ostomy

H. Partial or complete dentures

I. Renal to include difficulty in urination, dysuria, dribbling, incontinence, urgency, frequency, infections, stones

J. Musculoskeletal to include pain or stiffness in joints, redness, swelling, limited ROM of joints, fatigue, weakness, pain in muscles, arthritis, fractures

K. Endocrine to include diabetes, thyroid condition, increase in thirst, appetite, urination, heat or cold intolerance

L. Hematopoietic to include anemia, bruising, previous transfusions, skin hemorrhages, petechiae

M. Reproductive to include lesions on or drainage from penis or vulva, rashes or irritations on penis or vulva, vaginal infections, venereal diseases, infertility, birth control used, sexual difficulties, age at menarche/menopause, regularity, amount, frequency, duration of menses, bleeding between periods, after intercourse, after menopause, number of pregnancies, live births, abortions, complications during pregnancies, LMP, lumps or pain in breasts, last Pap smear, breast exam

N. Psychiatric to include depression, nervousness, mood swings, insomnia, self-concept, effect of stress, thoughts of suicide

# ■ Safety Assessment

**DEFINITION:** The collection of a data base concerning environmental, physical, and mental safety to be used in identifying nursing problems

## I. Interview for and record past history:
 A. Environmental factors affecting health status (air, hazardous occupation, water, vectors of disease)
 B. Kinds of accidents and injuries, accident proneness
 C. Safety aids in home or need for them

## II. Assess for:
 A. How safe patient feels in hospital
 B. Environmental factors such as cleanliness, arrangement of unit furniture and equipment, frayed wires or loose electrical connections, grounding where needed, floor free from articles or spilled liquids, contaminated material in or out of wastebasket or proper receptacle, equipment in need of repair, isolation and $O_2$ warning signs posted, bathroom facilities with safety bars for holding, lighting, temperature
 C. Bed in low position, side rails up or down as needed, call light in place within reach, articles within reach, wastebasket within reach, ash tray if needed, foot stool if needed
 D. Ability to protect self from harm
 E. Ability to perform daily functions and ambulation without assistance or amount of assistance needed
 F. Physical factors such as restraints, medications that affect mobility, breaks in skin, weakness, binders, eye shields, casts, IVs, gastric decompression, $O_2$, catheter, traction, isolation precautions or reverse isolation, pain, dressings
 G. Mental factors such as sensory impairment and use of glasses, hearing aid, vertigo, disoriented, level of consciousness, fear, anxiety, mistrust, confusion

## III. Administer:
 A. Medications as ordered (5 rights, identification—check $\times 3$)
 B. Treatments as ordered utilizing principles of safety

## IV. Perform/Provide:
 A. Identification of chart and records
 B. Identification of patient preceding any medication or treatment by armband

C. Correct use of addressograph for charts, requisitions, charges
D. Assistance in daily functions, ambulation, smoking as needed
E. Disposal of hazardous material properly
F. Isolation and reverse isolation precautions
G. Positioning and body alignment
H. Side rails, assistance to chair or stretcher
I. Restraints as ordered following principles of safety
J. Safe care of clothing, valuables, dentures, etc.
K. Special signs or warnings on door ($O_2$, levels of precautions)
L. All treatments and care utilizing medical asepsis or sterile techniques as required
M. All items, such as call light, water, tissues, wastebasket, within reach
N. Bed in low position unless otherwise indicated
O. Quick response to call light
P. Honest answers to questions

## V. Teach patient/family:
A. How to use call light, TV, bed adjustment
B. Route of evacuation for fire or other disaster

# ■ Diagnostic Procedures

**DEFINITION:** Procedures done to assist in medical diagnosis. May be done in radiology or nuclear medicine departments, special labs, or on the unit

**CONCEPT/NEED:** Anxiety

**NURSING DIAGNOSIS:** Anxiety related to lack of knowledge about procedure

**GOAL:** Reduced anxiety as evidenced by: verbalization, pulse WNL, ability to sleep at night

| INTERVENTION | RATIONALE |
|---|---|
| **I. Monitor, record, describe:** | |
| A. TPR, BP before procedure | A. Provides a baseline for comparison |
| **II. Assess for:** | |
| A. Other medical conditions and how test can affect them | A. May be contraindicated |
| B. Need for informed signed consent. Whether procedure was explained | B. For legal purposes, and to insure understanding |
| C. Other tests ordered and if interferences among tests exist | C. May cause tests to be repeated |
| D. Allergies to dyes, antibiotics, novacaine, shellfish | D. Insures patient safety |
| E. Contraindication to procedure or precautions such as pregnancy or restlessness | E. Insures patient safety |
| F. Equipment or supplies needed pre- or post-testing | F. Insures patient safety |
| G. Knowledge of procedure | G. ↓ anxiety |

### III. Administer:

A. Medications necessary to prepare for procedure as ordered or according to hospital policy

A. Necessary for accurate test results

B. Special diets, fluids in preparation given or withheld during procedure

B. Necessary for accurate test results

### IV. Perform/Provide:

A. Personal hygiene care before procedure with clothing for warmth and comfort

A. For patient comfort

B. Information to labs or departments regarding allergies, pregnancy, medical conditions, stability, NPO status, and need for medications and dietary requirements

B. Insures procedures being done correctly

C. Preparation such as enemas or other

C. Necessary for accurate test results

D. Removal of valuables, dentures, hair pins and give opportunity to void

D. Prevents loss. Bladder contents may cause discomfort

E. Assistance with transportation by chair, stretcher

E. Insures patient safety

F. Check chart for consent, lab results, physical exam if required

F. Insures patient safety

G. Preparation of room for patient's return including supplies and/or equipment needed

G. Insures patient safety

H. VS, diet, fluid, medications following procedure according to assessment of needs and orders

H. Insures identification of complications quickly

I. Information regarding when test results and implications will be available

I. ↓ anxiety

J. Time for questions and expression of concerns

J. ↓ anxiety

## V. Teach patient/family:

A. What is included in preparation for procedure and what is expected of patient

A. ↓ anxiety, insures cooperation

B. What will take place during procedure, to answer any questions, or reinforce physician explanation

B. ↓ anxiety

C. With use of written information about procedure

C. Reinforces teaching

D. No food or drink after midnight before procedure

D. Insures GI tract is empty. Threat to airway

E. Clarification of information if misunderstood

E. ↓ anxiety

F. Time scheduled for procedure

F. ↓ anxiety

G. Amount of time away from unit

G. ↓ anxiety

H. What will take place when returned to room

H. ↓ anxiety

# ■ Laboratory Tests/Specimen Collection

**DEFINITION:** Tests done on blood, urine, stool, body fluids, secretions, and discharges. Depending on the specimen or test ordered, examination is done in the laboratory department or on the unit

**CONCEPT/NEED:** Anxiety

**NURSING DIAGNOSIS:** Anxiety related to lack of information about procedure

**GOAL:** Reduced anxiety as evidenced by: verbalization, pulse WNL, ability to sleep at night

| INTERVENTION | RATIONALE |
|---|---|
| **II. Assess for:** | |
| A. Need for informed signed consent | A. For legal purposes, to insure understanding |
| B. Other conditions, interferences, or contraindications to the test | B. May cause serious complications |
| C. Equipment and supplies needed to collect specimen | C. Insures proper collection |
| D. Knowledge of procedure and why being done | D. ↓ anxiety |
| **III. Administer:** | |
| A. Medications before and during test | A. Necessary for accurate test results |
| B. Special fluids or foods in preparation for or during test | B. Necessary for accurate test results |
| **IV. Perform/Provide:** | |
| A. Identification of patient | A. Insures safety |
| B. Lab slip/requisition with accurate name and information | B. Prevents repetition |
| C. Accurate labeling of specimen | C. Prevents repetition of test or results of wrong patient |

D. Testing of urine, blood, or stool as ordered and record on flow sheet

D. May be done in unit

E. Assistance to physician collecting specimen

E. Insures accuracy

F. Collection of specimen and sending to lab immediately

F. Insures accuracy

G. Information regarding when test results will be available for physician to discuss with patient

G. ↓ anxiety

## V. Teach patient/family:

A. What will be done and why it is being done

A. ↓ anxiety

B. NPO after midnight if required

B. Need to repeat test

C. When specimen will be collected

C. Need to repeat test

D. Responsibility to save urine or stool and call nurse

D. Insures compliance

E. Who will collect specimen

E. ↓ anxiety

F. Test own specimen if applicable

F. Insures compliance

# ■ Pre-Operative Care

**DEFINITION:** The period of time between the time that surgery is planned and the time that surgery takes place. Special interventions are planned and carried out to assure physical and emotional safety before and following the procedure

**CONCEPT/NEED:** Anxiety

**NURSING DIAGNOSIS:** Anxiety related to loss of control, death

**GOAL:** Reduced anxiety as evidenced by: verbalization, pulse WNL, ability to sleep at night

| INTERVENTION | RATIONALE |
|---|---|
| **II. Assess for:** | |
| A. Feelings and concerns about surgery | A. ↓ anxiety |
| B. Basis of anxiety | B. Identifies how patient copes |
| C. Knowledge of procedure and purpose | C. ↓ anxiety |
| D. Knowledge of physical preparation | D. ↓ anxiety |
| E. Knowledge of what to expect following surgery | E. ↓ anxiety |
| **III. Administer:** | |
| A. Antianxiety medications as ordered | A. ↓ anxiety |
| **IV. Perform/Provide:** | |
| A. Time to verbalize fears and anxieties | A. ↓ anxiety |
| B. Acceptance without being judgmental, giving options | B. Allows for full expression |
| C. Nursing history and care plan involving patient | C. Needed for data base |
| D. Clergy if desired | D. ↓ anxiety |

## V. Teach patient/family:

A. Additional information about purpose and the procedure to be performed as reinforcement to physician

A. ↓ anxiety

B. Importance of informed consent

B. For legal purposes, to ensure knowledge of patient

C. About equipment in room, use of side rails, call light

C. Insures safety

D. Reasons for pre-operative treatments, enema, NPO, NG tube, IV, lab tests, catheter, medications

D. ↓ anxiety

E. Stay in recovery room, reason and how long

E. Varies according to surgical procedure

F. Medications will be given for pain

F. ↓ anxiety

G. Length of time in surgery

G. ↓ anxiety

H. Location of incision and possible size

H. ↓ anxiety

I. Ask questions or for explanations

I. ↓ anxiety

---

**CONCEPT/NEED:** Learning
Transport/Circulation

**NURSING DIAGNOSIS:** Knowledge deficit related to pulmonary/circulatory complications

**GOAL:** Knowledge deficit will decrease as evidenced by: performing leg exercises, turning, coughing, deep breathing

## INTERVENTION

## RATIONALE

### II. Assess for:

A. Cardiac/pulmonary status

A. Indicates circulation/oxygenation

B. Blood type and cross-match

B. Needed for blood transfusion

C. VS

C. Indicates circulatory status

## IV. Perform/Provide:

A. Removal of nail polish from fingernails — A. Observe for capillary refill

B. Turning, coughing, deep breathing — B. ↓ pooling of secretions

C. Ambulation with assistance — C. ↑ circulation

D. Information that VS will be taken frequently following surgery — D. ↓ anxiety

E. Information that O₂ may be given post-operatively — E. ↓ anxiety

F. How to use Triflow, blow bottles, IPPB — F. Insures patient compliance

---

**CONCEPT/NEED:** Nutrition
Fluid balance

**NURSING DIAGNOSIS:** Potential fluid volume deficit related to abnormal fluid loss. Potential alteration in nutrition: less than body requirements related to NPO

**GOAL:** Fluid balance will be maintained as evidenced by: good skin turgor, output of 50 cc/hr. Nutritional status will be maintained as evidenced by: IV during surgery

## IV. Perform/Provide:

A. Start IV with ordered fluids — A. Insures hydration

## V. Teach patient/family:

A. Reason for IV fluids and continuation post-operatively — A. ↓ anxiety

B. Why NPO important before surgery — B. Assures patient compliance

---

**CONCEPT/NEED:** Skin integrity/Personal hygiene

**NURSING DIAGNOSIS:** Impairment of skin integrity related to immobility/wound infection

**GOAL:** Skin integrity will be maintained as evidenced by: no redness, no swelling, skin clean and smooth

## IV. Perform/Provide

| | |
|---|---|
| A. Skin preparation if ordered | A. ↓ chance of infection |
| B. Shower with antibacterial soap if ordered | B. ↓ chance of infection |
| C. Morning care on day of surgery | C. ↑ comfort |

## V. Teach patient/family:

| | |
|---|---|
| A. Importance of movement in bed post-op | A. ↓ pain after surgery |
| B. Importance of not touching dressings | B. ↓ chance of infection |
| C. Reason for skin preparation | C. ↓ anxiety |

# ■ Post-Operative Care

**DEFINITION:** The period of time post-recovery room in which interventions are planned and carried out to return the patient to his or her normal functioning as safely and comfortable as possible

**CONCEPT/NEED:** Oxygenation

**NURSING DIAGNOSIS:** Ineffective breathing pattern related to restricted/diminished chest movement

**GOAL:** Breathing pattern will be maintained as evidenced by: patent airway, ABGs WNL, respirations 16–20/min, deep, regular rate, skin color—pink

## INTERVENTION

**I. Monitor, describe, record:**
   A. Respiration rate, depth and skin color q 30 min for 2 hr, then q 3–4 hr as needed
   B. Breath sounds q 2–4 hr, then q 24 hr as needed

**II. Assess for:**
   A. Potential lung complications such as infection, respiratory failure, laryngospasm
   B. Special interventions if procedure done involves respiratory system, e.g., pneumonectomy, lobectomy, atelectasis, emphysema

**III. Administer:**
   A. O₂, IPPB, Triflow, Mini Neb, as ordered and observe response

## RATIONALE

A. Assures oxygenation

B. Assures oxygenation

A. Pooling of secretions leads to infection

B. Need to monitor more closely

A. ↑ oxygenation

## IV. Perform/Provide:

| INTERVENTION | RATIONALE |
|---|---|
| A. Turning, coughing, deep breathing q 2 hr for 24 hr when awake, then q 4 hr | A. ↑ $O_2$ |
| B. Postural drainage if ordered | B. Aids in removal of secretions |
| C. Positioning to allow for chest expansion and ventilation, head to side if vomiting | C. ↑ $O_2$ |
| D. Suctioning (oropharyngeal) if mucus present, characteristics | D. Necessary if patient cannot raise secretions |
| E. Ambulation when possible and progress as indicated | E. ↓ venous stasis |

---

**CONCEPT/NEED:** Transport/Circulation

**NURSING DIAGNOSIS:** Alteration in tissue perfusion related to blood loss

**GOAL:** Adequate tissue perfusion as evidenced by: pulse rate—60–90 bpm, regular, no bleeding, skin warm, BP WNL

| INTERVENTION | RATIONALE |
|---|---|
| **I. Monitor, describe and record:** | |
| A. Pulse rate and quality, and BP q 30 min × 4, then q 4 hr for 4 days | A. For detection of hypotension |
| B. Skin and nail bed color, condition, temperature | B. Indicates circulatory status |
| **II. Assess for:** | |
| A. Special interventions if procedure done involves circulatory system, e.g., vein ligation, angina pectoris, hypertension | A. Chance of complications |
| B. Bleeding and other S&S of shock | B. Chance of hemorrhage |

C. Positive Homan's sign

D. Local warmth, swelling, pain, redness in legs

C. Indicates deep vein thrombosis

D. Indicates superficial vein thrombosis

### III. Administer:
A. Blood or blood components as ordered, or IV fluids

A. Combats hypovolemia

### IV. Perform/Provide:
A. Antiembolic hose

B. Exercises in bed, quadriceps, gluteal

C. Ambulation when possible and progress as indicated

A. ↓ venous pooling

B. ↑ circulation

C. ↑ circulation

---

**CONCEPT/NEED:** Pain

**NURSING DIAGNOSIS:** Alteration in comfort: pain related to incision

**GOAL:** Increased comfort as evidenced by: verbalization, VS WNL, no grimacing, ability to sleep at night

### INTERVENTION

### RATIONALE

### I. Monitor, describe, record:
A. VS q 4 hr or as needed

B. Pain characteristics and need for medication q 3–4 hr

C. Amount and quality of rest and sleep
(See Rest/Sleep Assessment, p. 35)

A. Indicates severity of pain

B. Needed for data base

C. Pain interferes with sleep

### II. Assess for:
A. Pressure on wound, e.g., cast, tight dressing

B. Nausea, vomiting causing pain

C. Overmedication leading to respiratory depression or hypotension

A. Determines pain area

B. Determines activity causing pain

C. May lead to serious complications

| | |
|---|---|
| D. Restlessness, irritability, fatigue | D. May indicate lack of rest |
| E. Response to or relief of pain following analgesic | E. Assures proper dosage to relieve pain |

### III. Administer:

| | |
|---|---|
| A. Analgesics as ordered/ needed | A. ↓ pain perception |
| B. Antiemetics as ordered/ needed | B. ↓ stimulation of vomiting center |

### IV. Perform/Provide:

| | |
|---|---|
| A. Pain relieving techniques (position change, back rub) | A. ↓ need for pain medications |
| B. Splinting wound when moving, coughing, ambulating | B. ↓ pain |
| C. Restful environment, noise and temperature control | C. ↓ pain perception |
| D. Schedule procedures around rest periods | D. Insures enough rest |

---

**CONCEPT/NEED:** Fluid balance

**NURSING DIAGNOSIS:** Fluid volume deficit related to inadequate oral intake

**GOAL:** Fluid balance will be maintained as evidenced by: good skin turgor, electrolytes WNL, I&O WNL

### INTERVENTION

### RATIONALE

#### I. Monitor, describe, record:

| | |
|---|---|
| A. I&O q 8 hr to include emesis, voiding, tube drainage | A. Insures proper fluid balance |
| B. IV infusion q 2–4 hr to include site, rate, type of fluid and patency | B. Detects extravasation |

C. Electrolytes (particularly $K^+$), BUN and urinalysis, and report abnormal levels to physician

C. May lead to serious complications

## II. Assess for:
A. History of renal disease

A. Needed for data base

B. Potential complications as result of renal function

B. May identify complications sooner

C. Special interventions if procedure done involves renal/genitourinary systems, e.g., nephrectomy, hysterectomy, cystitis

D. Patency and connections of all tubes and drains

D. Insures safety

E. Voiding within 6–8 hr

E. Identifies urinary retention

F. S&S of fluid imbalance (retention or loss) and report to physician

F. Identifies complications early

## III. Administer:
A. IV replacement fluids and electrolytes as ordered

A. Insures fluid and electrolyte balance

B. Electrolyte supplements PO when indicated or ordered

B. Insures fluid and electrolyte balance

## IV. Perform/Provide:
A. Catheterization if needed

A. Empties bladder

B. Daily weight at same time, scale, clothing if needed

B. Indicative of fluid status

C. Palpation of bladder for pain, distention q 4–8 hr

C. May indicate urinary retention

D. Fluid intake according to calculated individual needs, by mouth as indicated

D. Insures proper hydration

---

**CONCEPT/NEED:** Elimination
Nutrition

**NURSING DIAGNOSIS:** Potential alteration in elimination: bowel, related to loss of peristalsis. Potential alteration in nutrition: less than body requirements related to anorexia, vomiting

**GOAL:** Adequate elimination as evidenced by: bowel sounds present, BM by 3 days post-op. Adequate nutrition as evidenced by: progression to regular diet or previous special diet

## INTERVENTION

**I. Monitor, describe, record:**
    A. Nausea, vomiting q 4 hr
    B. Abdominal bowel sounds/ distention q 2–4 hr as needed
    C. Flatus and first BM post-op

**II. Assess for:**
    A. Potential complications to include constipation, impaction, diarrhea, paralytic ileus
    B. Special interventions if procedure involves the gastrointestinal system, e.g., cholecystectomy, hepatitis, colostomy
    C. Nasogastric or drainage tube patency, suctioning, drainage
    D. Bleeding in stools (occult or obvious) or emesis
    (See Gastrointestinal Assessment, p. 215)

**III. Administer:**
    A. Antiemetic as ordered

    B. Suppository/laxative/enema as ordered
    C. Antacids PO or NG tube as ordered, indicated

**IV. Perform/Provide:**
    A. Irrigation of NG tube
    B. pH of NG drainage

## RATIONALE

A. Fluid/electrolyte imbalance
B. No food is allowed until bowel sounds return

C. Indicates peristalsis

A. May identify complications early

B. Need to monitor more closely

C. Needed for proper draining

D. Indicates serious blood loss

A. Controls vomiting, protects airway
B. For proper elimination

C. ↓ gastric acidity

A. Maintains tube patency
B. Determines acidity of stomach contents

C. Hemoccult of drainage

D. Maintenance of NPO per assessment and orders

E. Diet progression as tolerated after bowel sounds return

C. Indicates GI bleeding

D. ↓ chance of paralytic ileus

E. ↓ trauma to GI tract

---

**CONCEPT/NEED:** Mobility/Activity

**NURSING DIAGNOSIS:** Activity intolerance related to incisional discomfort

**GOAL:** Activity will increase as evidenced by: progressive ambulation, ROM, ability to perform daily functions

## INTERVENTIONS

I. **Monitor, describe, record:**
   A. Active ROM
   B. Immobilization by cast or traction
   C. Amount and ability of movement in bed, chair, walking
   D. Type of assistance needed
   E. Decreased sensation
   F. Amount of self-care

II. **Assess for:**
   A. Potential complications of immobility
      (See Musculoskeletal Assessment, p. 301)
   B. Usual pattern, kind and amount of activity
   C. Special interventions if the procedure involves the musculoskeletal system, e.g., total hip replacement, laminectomy

## RATIONALE

A. Evaluates degree of immobility
B. Evaluates degree of immobility

C. Evaluates degree of immobility

D. Assists in planning care
E. Indicative of nerve damage
F. Assists in planning care

A. Insures safety

B. Assists in planning care

C. May need specific intervention

## III. Perform/Provide:

| | |
|---|---|
| A. Passive ROM as needed | A. ↑ tone, ↑ circulation |
| B. Proper body alignment | B. ↓ pressure areas |
| C. Repositioning as needed | C. ↓ pressure areas |
| D. Assistance with ambulation and daily functions as needed | D. Insures safety |
| E. Cast/traction care if applicable | E. Insures proper circulation |

---

**CONCEPT/NEED:** Skin integrity

**NURSING DIAGNOSIS:** Impairment of skin integrity related to immobility

**GOAL:** Absence of skin breakdown as evidenced by: no redness, no swelling, skin warm and dry

## INTERVENTION

## RATIONALE

### I. Monitor, describe, record:

A. Temperature q 4 hr as needed

A. Indicates infection

### II. Assess for:

A. Complications of wound closure or infection

A. May need rapid intervention

B. Special interventions if procedure done involves integumentary system, e.g., basal cell carcinoma, skin graft

B. Need to monitor more closely

C. Dressings, drains (amount, color, consistency, odor, patency)

C. May identify infection

D. Swelling, heat, redness of wound
(See Integumentary Assessment, p. 397)

D. Indicates infection

**III. Administer:**
    A. Antibiotics as ordered and observe for side effects     A. For infection

**IV. Perform/Provide:**
    A. Dressing changes or reinforcement as needed using sterile technique     A. Chance of infection

    B. Personal hygiene care QD     B. ↑ circulation to all areas, provides feeling of well-being

    C. Encouragement of dietary and fluid requirements to promote wound healing     C. Protein, vitamin C aids healing

# ■ Discharge Planning

**DEFINITION:** The planning that begins on admission of the patient and subsequent teaching that takes place before discharge from the hospital or agency

**CONCEPT/NEED:** Learning

**NURSING DIAGNOSIS:** Knowledge deficit related to treatment regimen necessary for home care

**GOAL:** Knowledge deficit will decrease as evidenced by: describing home treatment, stating changes that will need to be made in the home

| INTERVENTION | RATIONALE |
|---|---|
| **II. Assess for:** | |
| A. Type or quantity of education completed | A. Needed for appropriate teaching |
| B. Ability to recall events (forgetfulness), and comprehend technical content | B. May need written information |
| C. Vocabulary level, simple, complex or technical words | C. As appropriate for level of patient |
| D. Ability to comprehend words | D. Needed for appropriate teaching |
| E. Ability to comprehend ideas | E. Needed for appropriate teaching |
| F. Length of attention span | F. Need to teach for appropriate amount of time |
| G. Learning disabilities | G. Needed for appropriate teaching |
| H. Interest in learning | H. Learning will not take place if disinterested |
| I. Readiness to learn | I. Learning will not take place if patient is not ready |
| J. Value of learning | J. Value affects whether learning will take place |
| K. Physical limitation to include vision, hearing, psychomotor coordination | K. Must be integrated in teaching. Special preparations may be needed |
| L. Insight into illness and acceptance of illness | L. If patient is denying illness, learning will not occur |

M. Coping mechanisms to deal with illness    M. If patient is unable to cope with illness, learning will not occur

N. Level of understanding of illness, treatments, medications, modification of life style patterns    N. Needed for compliance of treatment

O. Necessary finances for implementation of plan    O. Needed for appropriate planning

P. Need for extended care facility or other placement    P. Needed for appropriate planning

Q. Usual life style patterns and habits to integrate into plan    Q. Needed for patient compliance

R. Home adjustments to be made    R. For discharge planning

## IV. Perform/Provide:

A. Mutually set goals for learning    A. ↑ compliance and feeling of independence

B. Lists of resources in community to use for continued care (pamphlets, booklets, pictures)    B. For patient's convenience

C. Information of S&S to report to physician    C. Provides early recognition of complications

D. Next appointment with physician    D. Provides continuity of care

E. Information on what to do in an emergency    E. ↓ anxiety

F. Information as to where to get equipment and supplies    F. For patient's convenience

G. Demonstration of procedures to be learned    G. Effective teaching tool

H. Emotional support and encouragement during learning    H. Enhances self-confidence

## V. Teach patient/family:

A. Special diet and restrictions    A. ↑ compliance

B. Medication self-administration with dosage, route, side effects, drug interactions, action of the drug    B. Insures patient safety

C. Tolerance for activity and special exercises
D. Fluid intake as indicated

E. Prevention of constipation
F. Rest periods
G. Refrain from taking OTC drugs without asking physician

H. Use of safety aids in walking, bathroom, steps
I. Skin and wound cleanliness
J. Ask questions when needed
K. Special teaching from each standard as appropriate to diagnosis

C. Prevents injury

D. Prevents dehydration or overhydration

E. For adequate elimination
F. For adequate rest/sleep
G. Prevents serious drug interactions

H. Prevents injury, facilitates daily functions
I. Prevents infection
J. Clarifies teaching
K. Individualizes teaching

# PSYCHOSOCIAL STANDARDS

- Psychosocial Assessment and Mental Status Examination
- Rest/Sleep Assessment
- Spiritual Assessment
- Work/Play/Recreation Assessment
- Anxiety Process
- Grieving Process

# ■ Psychosocial Assessment and Mental Status Examination

**DEFINITION:** The collection of a data base concerning all areas of mental health that may be used to identify nursing problems

## I. Interview for:

A. Past history

1. Childhood—what parents may have told patient

   a. Eating habits—allergies, likes/dislikes, finicky eater
   b. Bowel habits/toilet training—to what degree is the patient concerned with neatness? Evaluate personal hygiene. Evaluate for symptoms of prolonged enuresis, habitual constipation, recurrent diarrhea. Evaluate whether patient feels restricted from discussing these
   c. Disorders in learning speech habits—stuttering, lisping, hesitancy, excessive hand gesturing, autistic terms, neologism. When did the patient first talk
   d. Ambulation—when did the patient first start ambulating
   e. Sleep habits—heavy or light, regular or irregular
   f. Discipline—who disciplined, what type of discipline
   g. Playmates—attitudes toward games and partners in them? Particularly close friend. What became of the relationship?
   h. Unusual childhood illnesses or injuries
   i. Reactions to starting school—adjustments or experiences
   j. Behavior problems—truancy, lying, stealing, seclusive tendencies, cruelty
   k. Other

2. Adolescence

   a. Age and onset of puberty—voice changes, shaving, menstruation
   b. Sleep habits—heavy or light, hours of sleep, nightmares/dreams
   c. Friendship patterns—feelings about close friends
   d. Dating patterns
   e. Sexual experiences—first encounter, masturbation, VD
   f. High school—reactions, adjustments, experiences
   g. Separation from family—adjustment, age when left home
   h. Legal difficulties—arrest, convictions

      i. Drug use—heroin, barbiturate, alcohol, cocaine, LSD, etc.
  3. Adulthood
    a. Educational history—education achievements, special honors
    b. Attitude toward competition and compromise—ambition
    c. Vocational history
    d. Sexual adjustment—heterosexual, bisexual, homosexual
    e. Courtships and marriages
    f. Parenthood—problem children, preferred child, miscarriages, siblings that die
    g. Military history
    h. Religious attitudes
    i. Hobbies
    j. Goals—difficulties to overcome, vocational/educational ambitions

B. Family history
  1. Current household—members in the household, describe by name, age, relationship (write in patient's own words)
  2. Mother and father—earliest memory of each parent or person that raised child (detailed description)
  3. Relationship with parents and siblings—feelings about family, birth order, who seemed to get most attention, discipline
  4. Psychiatric history of family—arguments, alcoholism, suicide, separation, divorce, incarceration, and hospitalization

C. Patient's psychiatric history
  1. Psychiatric treatments, therapists, institutions—include discharge dates, permission to contact therapists, attitude toward past treatment
  2. Drugs prescribed—reason, responses, and side effects. OTC medicines and street drugs used. Drinking habits and amount of alcohol consumed (double the figure an alcoholic gives)
  3. Suicide potential—risk is greatest in adolescence and after 55. Also in chronic illness and with significant losses

D. History of present illness
  1. Current problems—most important, record events that led to problems

## II. Assess for:
A. General appearance—personal hygiene, clothing, physical characteristics, posture, gait, mannerisms, behavior during interview, age, facial expression, cosmetic use, gestures
B. Communication—tone, quality, flow, speed. Use of the following:

associative looseness, flight of ideas, blocking, circumstantiality, mutism, perseveration, word salad, echolalia

C. Emotion—mood, affect
D. Orientation—time, place, person
E. Memory/attention—recent, remote, inability to concentrate
F. Intellectual level—vocabulary level, abstract thinking, judgment, perception, insight
G. Thought content/perceptions—delusions, hallucinations, illusions

# ■ Rest/Sleep Assessment

**DEFINITION:** The collection of a data base concerning the areas of rest and sleep that may be used to identify nursing problems

**I. Interview for and record present history:**
- A. Usual sleeping patterns, times of retiring and awakening, heavy or light
- B. Hour of sleep/night
- C. Naps—frequency, times, length
- D. Aides used—prescriptions, OTC drugs, snacks, reading, walking
- E. Effectiveness of sleeping aids
- F. Conditions conducive to rest or sleep
- G. Environmental factors patient considers restful
- H. Beliefs about sleep needs
- I. Presence of pain to include type, character, duration, location precipitating/alleviating factors
- J. Dreams/nightmares

# ■ Spiritual Assessment

**DEFINITION:** The collection of a data base concerning spiritual needs that may be used to identify nursing problems

**I. Interview for and record past history:**
  A. Feelings about a supreme being and how this view deals with illness
  B. Feelings about what will happen during hospitalization/illness
  C. Specific people helpful in religious life
  D. Specific religious practices observed and degree of importance
    1. Dietary restrictions/preferences
    2. Symbols of importance—prayer, Bible, rosary, literature
    3. Ways of dealing with spiritual needs (wish to see priest, minister, rabbi, going to chapel)
    4. Rituals of importance—Sacrament of the Sick, Communion, Sabbath candles
  E. Religious restrictions dealing with health care
    1. Catholic—fasting, dietary rules
    2. Jewish—fasting, dietary laws, Sabbath
    3. Jehovah's Witness—blood transfusions
    4. Christian Scientist—medical treatment
    5. Islam—dietary laws
    6. Buddhism—vegetarian diet only
  F. Relationship of patient's beliefs to hospitalization/illness
  G. View of the dying patient (only if patient is terminal)
    1. Knowledge of prognosis
    2. Wish for clergy
    3. Treatment of body after death

# ■ Work/Play/Recreation Assessment

**DEFINITION:** The collection of a data base concerning work, play, and recreation that may be used to identify nursing problems

## I. Interview for and record past history:
A. Type of past employment
B. Feelings about past employment
C. Effects on health
D. Reasons for leaving

## II. Interview for and record present history:
A. Type of present employment
B. Feelings about work
C. Activity involved in work
D. Effect of environment on health (chemical, stressful)
E. Plans for returning to work
F. Housekeeping tasks, amount, kind, and done by whom
G. Need for more education or wish for retraining
H. Type, frequency, and degree of participation in play/recreation
I. Effect of illness on recreational interests
J. Substitute interests while illness is present
K. Need to change recreation permanently

# ■ Anxiety Process

**DEFINITION:** An emotional state (apprehension or dread) resulting from a known or unknown source of danger or threat. May be mild, moderate, acute or panic state

II. **Assess for:**
   A. Mild level of anxiety (e.g., increase in respirations, pulse, nausea, urge to urinate, stomach butterflies, sweaty palms, insomnia, irritability, fidgeting, headache, anorexia)
   B. Moderate level of anxiety (e.g., tachypnea, tachycardia, diarrhea, constipation, diaphoresis, nailbiting, foot swinging, pitch in voice changes, muscle tension, shaky voice, concentration on task only, withdrawal, crying)
   C. Acute level of anxiety (e.g., headache, muscle spasm and tension, sighing, dyspnea, dizziness, heartburn and belching, anorexia, impotence, frigidity, palpitations, tachycardia)
   D. Panic state (e.g., cold perspirations, trembling, hyperventilation, weakness, faintness, inability to concentrate, inability to speak, immobility, feeling of falling apart)
   E. Use of defense mechanisms
   F. Ability to perform daily functions and maintain interpersonal relationships

III. **Administer:**
   A. Antianxiety medications as ordered and note response
   B. Sedatives and hypnotics for insomnia as ordered

IV. **Perform/Provide:**
   A. Calm, quiet environment with recognition of level of anxiety
   B. Establish trusting nurse–patient relationship
   C. Listen and answer questions without judgments
   D. Avoid threatening experiences
   E. Give information on care, treatments, medications, procedures
   F. Assist to identify anxiety and causes
   G. Allow expression of feelings and behaviors
   H. Diversional activities, visiting, TV, reading, guided imagery, games
   I. Relaxation techniques
   J. Interact in a calm, confident, reassuring manner
   K. Acceptance of use of defense mechanisms and/or new methods of dealing with anxiety
   L. Feedback for attempts at new behaviors and effectiveness
   M. Someone to remain with patient

# ■ Grieving Process

**DEFINITION:** The reaction or emotional response to the actual or anticipated loss of a person, body part, or thing that is greatly valued

## II. Assess for:
   A. Feelings of fatigue, anxiety, sadness, anger, alienation from others, guilt, worthlessness, emptiness, anguish
   B. Behaviors such as loss of appetite or interest in appearance, crying, withdrawal, blaming, flattened affect, repetitive speech, irritation with others
   C. Coping mechanisms used and stage of grief

## III. Administer:
   A. Antidepressant as ordered and note response

## IV. Perform/Provide:
   A. Allowance for expression of feelings and listen attentively
   B. Privacy
   C. Willingness to be present and to help
   D. Acceptance of the grief and behaviors exhibited
   E. Support without confrontation
   F. Assurance that feelings and behaviors are normal and expected
   G. Time to view loss (in cases of body part) and support when ready
   H. Assistance to adapt to change in life style because of loss, accept reality
   I. Independence in carrying out care and responsibilities with encouragement

# NEUROLOGICAL SYSTEM STANDARDS

- Neurological System Assessment
- Brain Tumor
- Cerebrovascular Accident
- Herniated Intervertebral Disk (Herniated Nucleus Pulposus)
- Intracranial Infections (Brain Abscess, Meningitis, Encephalitis)
- Seizure Disorders

# ■ Neurological System Assessment

**DEFINITION:** The collection of a data base concerning the neurological system and its functional capabilities to be used in identifying nursing problems related to this system

I. **Interview for and record past history:**
   A. Previous neurological or sensory conditions such as seizures, headaches, dizziness
   B. Family members with neurological conditions related to the neuro-system
   C. Previous operations, injuries, or chronic conditions related to the neuro-system
   D. Behavioral changes, confusion, disorientation, emotional changes
   E. Allergies and immunizations
   F. Infections, seizure disorders, head injuries
   G. Drug and alcohol abuse

II. **Interview for present history:**
   A. Chief complaint
   B. Onset and length of illness
   C. Knowledge of disease, procedures, and planned therapy
   D. Medications taken for neurological problems
   E. Results of CBC, ABGs, electrolytes, enzymes, cerebrospinal fluid analysis, gastric analysis with histamine, EEG, myelogram, lumbar puncture, brain scan, CAT scan

III. **Inspection for:**
   A. Gait, coordination, balance
   B. Tremors, resting or intention
   C. Ataxia, speech difficulty, difficulty swallowing
   D. Symmetry of muscle size, loss of muscle mass
   E. Muscle tone—spasticity, flaccidity, uncoordination
   F. Muscle strength—upper and lower extremities
   G. Involuntary muscle movements—tics, fasciculation
   H. Test the cranial nerves
      1. Olfactory (smell)—identifies odors, coffee, alcohol
      2. Optic (visual fields)—gross confrontation test, wiggle fingers. Visual acuity—Snellen eye chart
      3. Oculomotor—pupil constriction. Accommodation—pupil change of near and far objects, movement of eye muscles

4. Trochlear—movement of eye muscle
5. Trigeminal—jaw muscle and muscle of mastication, open and close jaw tightly. Ophthalmic, maxillary, and mandibular—identify sharp and dull sensation on each area with eyes closed
6. Abducens—movement of eye muscle
7. Facial—movement of muscles of face and scalp, grimacing, close eyes. Taste—identify familiar tastes, coffee, sugar
8. Acoustic–cochlear—Weber/Rinne tests. Vestibular—Romberg test
9. Glossopharyngeal—pain, temperature in throat and pharynx, not usually done
10. Vagus—sensation in larynx, trachea, lungs. Esophagus—gag reflex, swallowing, phonation
11. Spinal accessory—muscles of head and upper shoulders—shrug shoulders against resistance and rotate head against resistance
12. Hypoglossal—tongue movements, protruding tongue, push tongue against cheek

# ■ Brain Tumor

**DEFINITION:** Temporal lobe, occipital, cerebellum, and parietal are areas where neoplasms may arise within the brain. These are divided into acoustic neuromas, meningiomas, pituitary adenomas, and gliomas

**CONCEPT/NEED:** Pain

**NURSING DIAGNOSIS:** Alteration in comfort: pain related to pressure

**GOAL:** Increased comfort as evidenced by: verbalization, reduced requests for pain medications

| INTERVENTION | RATIONALE |
|---|---|
| I. **Monitor, describe, record:** | |
| A. Pain, duration, radiation, intensity, quality | A. Needed for data base |
| B. Effectiveness of pain relief | B. Use conservative treatment first |
| C. LOC | C. Identifies complications |
| III. **Administer:** | |
| A. Analgesics as ordered | A. Relieves pain |
| IV. **Perform/Provide:** | |
| A. Change position slowly and gradually | A. Prevents pain |
| B. Elevate head of bed 15 degrees | B. Promotes comfort |
| C. Pain relief measure that patient suggests | C. ↑ confidence and independence |
| D. Bedrest while pain is occurring | D. Promotes comfort |
| E. Guided imagery or relaxation techniques | E. ↓ pain |

**CONCEPT/NEED:** Safety

**NURSING DIAGNOSIS:** Potential physical injury related to falls

**GOAL:** Injuries will be prevented as evidenced by: no falls

| INTERVENTION | RATIONALE |
|---|---|
| II. **Assess for:** | |
|     A. Neurological status to include LOC, pupil response, reflexes | A. Needed for data base |
| III. **Administer:** | |
|     A. Restraints as needed | A. For confused patient |
| IV. **Perform/Provide** | |
|     A. Orientation to surroundings if patient's sight is affected | A. Insures safety |
|     B. Institute seizure precautions to include padded bedrails, pillow under head, insert oral airway, q 15 min checks, quiet environment | B. Insures safety |
|     C. Orientation as needed | C. Presents reality |
|     D. Night light on in bathroom | D. ↓ confusion |
|     E. Call bell within easy reach | E. Insures safety |

# ■ Cerebrovascular Accident

**DEFINITION:** A condition in which blood flow is obstructed in the brain due to cerebral thrombosis, cerebral hemorrhage, cerebral embolism

**CONCEPT/NEED:** Oxygenation

**NURSING DIAGNOSIS:** Ineffective breathing pattern related to obstruction

**GOAL:** Adequate breathing pattern as evidenced by: respiration WNL, adequate skin color

## INTERVENTION

I. **Monitor, describe, record:**
   A. Respiration rate, depth, skin color q 2–4 hr
   B. Breath sounds q 2–4 hr

II. **Assess for:**
   A. Skin color, skin temperature

III. **Administer:**
   A. $O_2$ or ventilation as ordered

IV. **Perform/Provide:**
   A. Turning, coughing, deep breathing q 2 hr
   B. Postural drainage as ordered
   C. Positioning to allow for chest expansion and ventilation, head to side to prevent aspiration if vomiting
   D. Suctioning of mucus if possible
   E. Ambulation when possible and progress as indicated

## RATIONALE

A. Indicates altered respiratory function
B. Indicates amount of aeration

A. Indicates aeration

A. Maintains oxygenation

A. Effective method of reducing secretions
B. ↓ secretions
C. ↑ aeration

D. Prevents aspiration, ↓ congestion

E. ↓ chance of pooling of secretions in the base of the lungs

**CONCEPT/NEED:** Transport/Circulation

**NURSING DIAGNOSIS:** Alteration in tissue perfusion related to obstruction

**GOAL:** Adequate tissue perfusion as evidenced by: adequate pulses throughout body, Glasgow Scale WNL

| INTERVENTION | RATIONALE |
|---|---|
| **I. Monitor, describe, record:** | |
| A. BP, pulse q 2 hr or more often if indicated | A. Good indicator of tissue perfusion and circulatory status |
| B. Intake and output q 8 hr | B. Decreased hydration may cause decreased blood flow to the brain |
| C. Skin color and nailbeds q 2 hr | C. Decreased color indicates poor peripheral blood flow |
| **II. Assess:** | |
| A. Neurological status q 1 hr including LOC, speech, orientation, pupil reactivity or use the Glasgow Scale | A. Prevents serious complications |
| **III. Administer:** | |
| A. IV fluids as ordered | A. Maintains adequate hydration |
| B. O₂ ventilation as ordered | B. Maintains oxygenation |
| C. Hyperbaric therapy when available | C. May increase O₂ to tissues |
| **IV. Perform/Provide:** | |
| A. ROM TID | A. Provides increased circulation |
| B. Reposition q 2 hr | B. Prevents blood pooling and hemostasis |

---

**CONCEPT/NEED:** Mobility/Immobility

**NURSING DIAGNOSIS:** Impaired physical mobility related to lack of sensation

**GOAL:** Adequate mobility as evidenced by: no contractures, ROM, progressive activity

| INTERVENTION | RATIONALE |
|---|---|

**I. Monitor, describe, record:**
- A. ROM of extremities — A. Promotes circulation and muscle tone

**II. Assess for:**
- A. Amount of disability QD — A. Needed for reassessment
- B. Amount of tasks that can be performed — B. Needed for reassessment

**III. Perform/Provide:**
- A. ROM of all extremities q 8 hr — A. Promotes circulation and muscle tone
- B. Alignment of body — B. Prevents pain and contractures
- C. Trochanter roll, place along affected thigh — C. ↓ external rotation and promotes functional position
- D. Support hand and arm higher than level of heart — D. Allows for drainage of fluid, ↓ edema
- E. Position change q 2 hr (turn on unaffected side) — E. ↓ hemostasis
- F. Elevate head of bed 15 degrees when patient is supine — F. ↓ chance of flexion contractures
- G. Assistance with ambulation as soon as possible — G. ↑ circulation and promotes muscle tone
- H. Footboard — H. Prevents footdrop

---

**CONCEPT/NEED:** Communication

**NURSING DIAGNOSIS:** Impaired verbal communication related to loss of speech

**GOAL:** Adequate communication as evidenced by: communication through written word

| INTERVENTION | RATIONALE |
|---|---|

**I. Monitor, describe, record:**
- A. Level of speech impairment, note on Kardex — A. Alerts other staff to patient's condition

**II. Assess for:**
- A. Degree of disability — A. Needed for data base

## III. Perform/Provide:
A. Alternate methods of communication

A. Helps to facilitate understanding patient's needs

B. Anticipate patient's needs

B. Helps to lower patient's anxiety

# ■ Herniated Intervertebral Disk (Herniated Nucleus Pulposus)

**DEFINITION:** May be caused by trauma. The result is a prolapse of the nucleus pulposus which lies between the vertebrae

**CONCEPT/NEED:** Pain

**NURSING DIAGNOSIS:** Alteration in comfort: pain related to inflammation

**GOAL:** Increased comfort as evidenced by: verbalization, absence of grimacing, ability to perform daily functions

## INTERVENTION

**I. Monitor, describe, record:**
- A. Pain, duration, radiation, intensity, quality
- B. Effectiveness of pain relief
- C. Identify lengths of legs

**III. Administer:**
- A. Analgesics/muscle relaxants as ordered

**IV. Perform/Provide:**
- A. Change position slowly and gradually
- B. Elevate head of bed 15 degrees
- C. Pain relief measure that patient suggests
- D. Bedrest while pain is occurring
- E. Guided imagery or relaxation techniques

## RATIONALE

- A. Needed for data base
- B. Use conservative treatment first
- C. Identifies disk rupture

- A. Relieves pain

- A. Prevents pain
- B. Promotes comfort
- C. ↑ confidence and independence
- D. Promotes comfort
- E. ↓ pain

F. Traction, pelvic
G. Physical therapy
H. Cervical collar/brace

V. **Teach patient/family:**
   A. Proper body mechanics
   B. Relaxation techniques

F. Relieves pressure on nerves
G. Relieves pressure
H. Corrects alignment

A. ↓ stress
B. Relieves pain

# ■ Intracranial Infections (Brain Abscess, Meningitis, Encephalitis)

**DEFINITION:** Meningitis is an inflammation of the meninges which cover the spinal cord. Encephalitis is an inflammation of the brain and the meninges. Both are serious disorders

**CONCEPT/NEED:** Oxygenation

**NURSING DIAGNOSIS:** Ineffective breathing pattern due to inflammation

**GOAL:** Normal breathing pattern as evidenced by: respirations WNL, absence of cyanosis

| INTERVENTION | RATIONALE |
|---|---|
| **I. Monitor, describe, record:** | |
| A. Respiration rate, depth, pattern, skin color q 2 hr | A. Indicates altered pattern |
| B. Breath sounds, airway patency q 2 hr | B. Indicates amount of aeration |
| C. VS q 4 hr | C. May indicate complication |
| D. Gag, swallow reflex q 1 hr | D. Needed to prevent aspiration |
| **II. Assess for:** | |
| A. Confusion, restlessness | A. Indicates decreased $O_2$ |
| B. Chest x-ray | B. May show consolidation |
| C. ABGs | C. $\downarrow O_2$ |
| **III. Administer:** | |
| A. $O_2$ as ordered | A. Maintains $O_2$ |
| **IV. Perform/Provide:** | |
| A. Turning, coughing and deep breathing q 2 hr | A. $\uparrow$ aeration |
| B. Postural drainage as ordered | B. Effective in reducing secretions |

| | |
|---|---|
| C. Positioning to allow for chest expansion and ventilation | C. ↑ $O_2$ |
| D. Suctioning of mucus if present | D. Prevents aspiration |
| E. Strict isolation until patient has been on antibiotics 24 hr | E. Considered infective until this time |

---

**CONCEPT/NEED:** Safety

**NURSING DIAGNOSIS:** Potential physical injury related to falls, infection

**GOAL:** Reduced potential for injury as evidenced by: no falls, infection

| INTERVENTION | RATIONALE |
|---|---|
| **II. Assess for:** | |
| A. Neurological status to include LOC, pupil responses, reflexes | A. Indicates complications |
| **III. Administer:** | |
| A. IV Valium or anticonvulsants | A. ↓ seizure threshold |
| B. Corticosteroids | B. ↓ inflammation |
| C. Antibiotics | C. Controls infection |
| **IV. Perform/Provide:** | |
| A. Seizure precautions (See Seizures, p. 54) | A. Prevents injury |
| **V. Teach patient/family:** | |
| A. Medications: time, purpose, side effects, dosage | A. Insures safety |
| B. Discuss prophylactic antibiotic treatment for family | B. Prevents contamination |
| C. Basic knowledge of disease process | C. ↓ anxiety |
| D. Proper handwashing and disposal of paper products containing infectious discharge | D. Prevents infection |

**CONCEPT/NEED:** Transport/Circulation

**NURSING DIAGNOSIS:** Alteration in tissue perfusion related to inflammation

**GOAL:** Adequate tissue perfusion as evidenced by: BP, pulse WNL

| INTERVENTIONS | RATIONALE |
|---|---|
| **I. Monitor, describe, record:** | |
|   A. BP, pulse q 2 hr | A. Indicates tissue perfusion |
|   B. I&O and ratio q 8 hr | B. Decreased blood flow will lower output |
|   C. Temperature q 4 hr | C. Indicates dehydration |
|   D. Skin color/nailbeds q 2 hr | D. Peripheral blood flow |
| **III. Administer:** | |
|   A. Corticosteroids | A. ↓ inflammation |
|   B. IV fluids as ordered | B. Maintains hydration |
| **IV. Perform/Provide:** | |
|   A. ROM TID | A. ↑ circulation |
|   B. Repositioning q 2 hr | B. Prevents hemostasis |

# ■ Seizure Disorders

**DEFINITION:** Seizures cause uncoordinated movements of the entire body. There are several types such as grand mal (tonic/clonic), petit mal, (absence attacks), focal-motor (Jacksonian), psychomotor (temporal lobe, limbic). The care included will have to be adapted to each specific type of seizure

**CONCEPT/NEED:** Oxygenation

**NURSING DIAGNOSIS:** Potential ineffective airway clearance related to obstruction

**GOAL:** Effective airway clearance as evidenced by: respirations 16–20, no cyanosis of lips

| INTERVENTION | RATIONALE |
|---|---|
| **I. Monitor, describe, record:** | |
| A. Respiration rate, depth, skin color q 2–4 hr | A. Indicates altered respiratory function |
| B. Breath sounds q 2–4 hr | B. Indicates amount of aeration |
| **II. Assess for:** | |
| A. Character, rate, depth of respirations | A. Needed for data base |
| B. Skin color, nailbeds | B. Indicates aeration |
| **III. Administer:** | |
| A. $O_2$ as ordered | A. Maintains oxygenation |
| **IV. Perform/Provide:** | |
| A. Suctioning of mucus if needed | A. Prevents aspiration and reduces congestion |
| B. Insertion of oral airway or rolled washcloth | B. Prevents decreased respirations |
| C. Loosen all clothing | C. Allows for adequate chest expansion |

**CONCEPT/NEED:** Safety

**NURSING DIAGNOSIS:** Potential physical injury related to falls

**GOAL:** Safety maintained as evidenced by: no falls

## INTERVENTION

II. **Assess for:**
   A. Neurological status to include LOC, pupils' response, reflexes

III. **Administer:**
   A. IV Valium or anticonvulsants as ordered

IV. **Perform/Provide:**
   A. Padded bedrails
   B. Insert oral airway or rolled washcloth
   C. Remove furniture near patient
   D. Remain with patient at all times
   E. Allow patient to seize without restricting movement
   F. Allow patient to slide to floor. Do not attempt to lift patient

## RATIONALE

A. Needed for data base

A. ↓ seizures

A. Insures safety
B. Prevents obstruction
C. Insures safety
D. Insures safety
E. Could harm patient if restrained
F. Prevents injury

# CARDIOVASCULAR SYSTEM STANDARDS

- Cardiovascular System Assessment
- Angina Pectoris
- Congestive Heart Failure
- Diminished Arterial Circulation to Extremities
- Hypertension
- Myocardial Infarction
- Thrombophlebitis/Venous Thrombosis
- Varicose Veins/Venous Insufficiency
- Vein Ligation/Stripping

# ■ Cardiovascular System Assessment

**DEFINITION:** The collection of a data base concerning the cardiovascular system and its functional capabilities to be used in identifying nursing problems related to transport/circulation

## I. Interview for and record past history:
A. Previous heart or blood vessel conditions such as hypertension, rheumatic fever, heart attack, leg ulcer, varicose veins, diabetes, obesity, heart surgery
B. Previous chest pain, pain in legs, heart palpitations, shortness of breath, ankle swelling, cold, numbness or tingling of arms or legs
C. Family members with heart or vein/artery conditions
D. Allergies and immunizations
E. Smoking, alcoholic drinks per day and years
F. Low cholesterol or salt-free diet
G. Cough with blood in sputum, wheezing
H. Sleeping with head elevated
I. Dizziness or fainting, indigestion, fatigue
J. Occupation, usual activity, sleep pattern
K. Usual pulse and blood pressure and factors that increase or decrease rate
L. Medications taken for heart condition, hypertension, vascular diseases, pain and response (prescribed and OTC)
M. Past ECG, arteriography, venography, x-ray or other blood tests and results and stress test

## II. Interview for and record present history:
A. Chief complaint
B. Onset, where took place, length of illness
C. Principal signs and symptoms
D. Knowledge of disease, procedures, and planned therapy
E. Results of ECG, x-ray, CBC, enzymes, scans, electrolytes, arteriography, venography, isoenzymes, ESR, cholesterol, PT, PTT, urinalysis, stress test, cardiac catheterization
F. $O_2$ and any other treatments
G. Medications taken for any cardiovascular problem

## III. Inspect for:
A. Symmetry of chest

B. Pulsations in the aortic area (2nd interspace, right of sternum), pulmonary area (2nd and 3rd interspaces on left), right ventricular area (lower half of sternum to the left), apical or left ventricular area (5th intercostal space at midclavicular line)

C. Point of maximum intensity (PMI) 2–3 cm in diameter at 5th interspace, 8 cm left of midsternal line in sitting or supine position

D. Symmetry of legs and arms

E. Arms, hands and legs, feet skin for color, texture (pink, smooth, warm, dry)

F. Hair distribution on legs and arms, clubbing of fingers

G. Rashes, scars, ulcers, exudate (brownish color, eschar, irregular shape for ulcerations and chronic venous stasis)

H. Veins even with skin surface or venous enlargement

I. Color change of extremities when dangling or elevated (should return to normal in 10 sec)

J. Trendelenburg test for vein valve competency (normal is filling from below, upward)

K. Capillary refill or nailbeds, less than 3 sec

## IV. Palpate for:

A. Skin of extremities smooth, dry, warm to touch

B. Masses in extremities and chest

C. Pain or tenderness in chest or extremities

D. Veins for smoothness and fullness, dilated tortuous veins

E. Cardiac thrills (pulsations of the heart that feel like the throat of a purring cat)

F. Radial pulse rate and characteristics

G. Femoral, popliteal, carotid, temporal, and dorsalis pedis pulses rate and characteristics

H. Apical pulse, PMI, other areas of pulsations of the heart

I. Edema in legs including pitting edema

J. Calf for signs of phlebitis (squeeze calf muscle and feel for tension of muscle noting tenderness)

K. Positive or negative Homan's sign

## V. Auscultate for:

A. Apical/radial pulse noting rate, regularity, and pulse deficit

B. Apical pulse noting rate, regularity, intensity

C. Blood pressure using brachial artery and noting Korotkoff phases and pulse pressure

D. Carotid artery for bruits

E. Aortic valve at 2nd intercostal space right of sternum noting rate, regularity, pitch, and intensity of S1, and S2 (S2 has higher pitch and greater intensity over aortic valve)

F. Pulmonic valve at 2nd intercostal space left of sternum noting rate, regularity, pitch, and intensity of S1 and S2 (S2 has higher pitch and greater intensity over pulmonic valve)

G. Tricuspid valve near lower left sternal border noting rate, regularity, pitch, and intensity of S1 and S2 (S1 has lower pitch and greater intensity over tricuspid valve)

H. Mitral valve (apical pulse) at 5th intercostal space at midclavicular line noting rate, regularity, pitch, and intensity of S1 and S2 (S1 has lower pitch and greater intensity over mitral valve)

I. S3 and S4 in children and note characteristics. Abnormal in adults

J. Murmur noting timing, location, sound distribution, location of maximum intensity, pitch (high, medium, low), and amplitude (faint, loud, very loud)

K. Clicks and snaps noting timing, intensity, and pitch

# ■ Angina Pectoris

**DEFINITION:** Substernal or precordial chest pain that may radiate to the left arm as a result of inadequate $O_2$ supply to the myocardium

**CONCEPT/NEED:** Transport/Circulation

**NURSING DIAGNOSIS:** Alteration in tissue perfusion: peripheral to myocardial vasoconstriction

**GOAL:** Tissue perfusion will be maintained as evidenced by: heart rate— 60–80 bpm, regular rhythm, skin color—pink, warm, dry

## INTERVENTION

**I. Monitor, describe, record:**
  A. Pulse, respirations, and characteristics q 4 hr
  B. Apical/radial pulse BID
  C. Peripheral pulses

  D. BP q 4 hr lying and standing both arms
  E. ECG

**II. Assess for:**
  A. S&S of complications

  B. Shortness of breath, cyanosis
  C. ECG and x-ray results (See Cardiovasulcar Assessment, p. 59)

**III. Administer:**
  A. $O_2$ as ordered
  B. Beta-adrenergic blocking agents or calcium blockers as ordered

## RATIONALE

A. Indicates circulatory status

B. Indicates circulatory status
C. Indicates circulation in extremities

D. May indicate orthostatic hypotension
E. May indicate MI, syncope, or convulsions

A. A large number of patients with angina pectoris develop an MI at a later date
B. Indicates impaired $O_2$ exchange

C. Reveals abnormalities such as narrowing or coronary vessels

A. For adequate $O_2$ to tissues
B. ↓ $O_2$ requirement of myocardium

C. Vasodilators as ordered

C. Dilates coronary vessels increasing blood flow to myocardium

## IV. Perform/Provide:
A. Rest periods
B. Comfortable, quiet environment
C. Position for comfort

A. ↓ need for $O_2$
B. Strong emotions increase heart's need for $O_2$
C. Eases breathing

## V. Teach patient/family:
A. Need not to smoke

B. Disease process and treatment

C. Restrictions in activity. Avoid heavy meals

D. Avoid cold temperatures (walk slowly, cover nose and mouth, dress warmly)

E. About diagnostic test and procedures

A. ↑ pulse and BP, and work of the heart

B. Helps prevent recurrence

C. Heavy exertion or meals increase need for $O_2$

D. Causes vasoconstriction and increases BP resulting in increased $O_2$ demand

E. Familiarity reduces anxiety

---

**CONCEPT/NEED:** Pain

**NURSING DIAGNOSIS:** Potential alteration in comfort: pain related to myocardial vasoconstriction

**GOAL:** Increased comfort as evidenced by: verbalization, no grimacing, ability to tolerate increased activity without pain

## INTERVENTION

## RATIONALE

### II. Assess for:
A. Characteristics of pain, squeezing, pressing, or aching. Retrosternal or left of sternum. Radiating to left shoulder, arm down to wrist and fingers or to neck and jaw. Duration of 5 min or longer

A. Pain of angina is never described as sharp. It is usually retrosternal. Pain is rarely localized and lasts less than 3 min, rarely more than 15–20 min

B. Associated symptoms of dyspnea, pallor, sweating, dizziness, faintness
C. How relieved
D. What precipitates pain

B. Symptoms associated with hypotension
C. Relieved by rest and nitroglycerin
D. A detailed history is the key to the diagnosis

## III. Administer:
A. Analgesics as ordered
B. Vasodilators (nitrates) as ordered

A. ↓ pain perception
B. Dilates coronary vessels increasing blood flow to myocardium

## IV. Perform/Provide:
A. Rest until pain subsides, planned rest to prevent episodes
B. Position of comfort
C. Comfortable, quiet environment

A. Angina usually follows pattern of exertion-pain-rest-relief. Decreases $O_2$ need
B. ↓ pain
C. Pain can be precipitated by increased emotion and excitement

## V. Teach patient/family:
A. Schedule rest and activity periods
B. Identify situations to avoid and when to take medications to prevent pain
C. Take drug as soon as pain begins. Carry at all times
D. Side effects such as headache, dizziness, and flushing
E. Method of administration by sublingual, topical, inhalation

F. Rest after taking drug. May repeat q 5–10 min ×3

G. Have fresh supply, not older than 6 months
H. Avoid OTC drugs

A. Avoid overexertion known to cause pain
B. Pain usually follows increased emotions, heavy eating, or exposure to cold
C. ↓ vasoconstriction immediately
D. May cause anxiety or unsafe ambulation
E. Proper route insures desired results

F. If pain is not relieved by rest and nitroglycerin, patient must seek medical help
G. Inactivated by air and time
H. May mask a serious problem or interact with OTC drugs

I. Report severe side effects to physician
J. Store drug in dark container at room temperature
K. May take prior to exertion (intercourse)

I. Medication may need to be changed or dose adjusted
J. Is inactivated by heat, moisture, and light
K. Causes vasodilation before exertion which reduces chance of pain

---

**CONCEPT/NEED:** Anxiety

**NURSING DIAGNOSIS:** Anxiety related to possible death

**GOAL:** Decreased anxiety as evidenced by: verbalization, pulse WNL, absence of flushing, sweating

## INTERVENTION

**II. Assess for:**
A. Verbal and nonverbal clues of anxiety

B. Personal resources to cope with stress
C. Responses to information and treatments
D. Changes in life style (See Psychosocial Assessment for further guidelines, p. 31)

**IV. Perform/Provide:**
A. Accepting environment to state feelings
B. Environment that avoids anxiety-producing situations

C. Referral for counseling for extremely anxious individual
D. Encouragement to perform self-care as able

## RATIONALE

A. Client may be unable to openly communicate. Open communication reduces stress
B. Provides emotional support

C. Treatments and information may increase or decrease anxiety
D. Role conflict may occur due to need for rest and reduced anxiety

A. Provides emotional support

B. Increase of adrenalin and BP with anxiety leading to increased heart rate, pain
C. May need professional psychiatric assistance
D. ↓ sense of helplessness and emotional trauma

## V. Teach patient/family:

A. Avoid anxiety-producing situations

B. Possible changes in patterns of living to include work if needed

A. ↓ vasoconstriction of myocardium

B. Changes may be needed to reduce anxiety

---

**CONCEPT/NEED:** Mobility/Activity

**NURSING DIAGNOSIS:** Activity intolerance related to exertion

**GOAL:** Activity tolerance will increase as evidenced by: participation in progressive exercise program

## INTERVENTION

### RATIONALE

## II. Assess for:

A. Activity, nutrition, and elimination patterns that precipitate symptoms

B. Changes in VS before and after activity

A. Detailed history is needed for proper diagnosis

B. Indicates myocardial status

## III. Administer:

A. Laxative or stool softener as ordered

A. Prevents constipation

## IV. Perform/Provide:

A. Planned rest and activity periods

B. Activity limited to level of fatigue or discomfort. ROM if needed

C. Rest after meals

D. Special diet as ordered (low calorie, low Na, or small feedings)

E. Fluid and dietary adjustments to prevent constipation

A. ↓ workload on heart

B. Regular graded exercise below the pain threshold increases circulation

C. ↓ stress on heart

D. Small feedings reduce anginal pain

E. Valsalva maneuver increases thoracic pressure, decreases venous return. Causes reflex bradycardia

# V. Teach patient/family:

A. Adherence to an exercise/activity regimen

A. Promotes circulation

B. Avoid lifting and pushing

B. ↑ $O_2$ demand resulting in pain

C. Avoid sexual activity unless rested and having taken medications

C. ↑ $O_2$ demand

D. Avoid overeating or large meals

D. ↑ heart rate, heavier demand on heart

E. Avoid caffeine drinks

E. ↑ heart rate

F. Maintain WT at an approved level

F. Obesity increases heart rate, and cardiac workload

G. Maintenance of bowel elimination pattern without straining

G. Valsalva maneuver places strain on heart, and stimulates parasympathetic nervous system

H. Diet restrictions of calories, Na, cholesterol

H. ↓ workload of heart

# ■ Congestive Heart Failure

**DEFINITION:** Reduced cardiac function leading to a low cardiac output resulting in a retention of fluid in the systemic (peripheral tissues) or pulmonary (lungs) circulation

**CONCEPT/NEED:** Oxygenation

**NURSING DIAGNOSIS:** Ineffective breathing pattern related to fluid accumulation

**GOAL:** Effective breathing pattern as evidenced by: use of accessory muscles for breathing, respirations deep and regular

| INTERVENTION | RATIONALE |
|---|---|
| **I. Monitor, describe, record:** | |
| A. Respirations q 4 hr | A. Dyspnea, sign of fatigue |
| B. Lung sounds. Rales are a common finding | B. Tachypnea is a sign of decreased $O_2$ (compensatory factor) |
| **II. Assess for:** | |
| A. Pulmonary status to include history and physical assessment | A. Needed for data base |
| B. Temperature q 4 hr | B. High temperature may indicate infection or pulmonary embolism |
| C. Neck vein distention | C. ↑ blood in pulmonary system |
| D. Restlessness, increased respirations, Cheyne-Stokes respirations | D. Symptom of decreased $O_2$ |
| E. Chest x-ray | E. Pulmonary congestion is shown |
| F. Arterial blood gases | F. Late sign, increased $P_{CO_2}$, decreased $P_{O_2}$ |
| G. Cough—hemoptysis and characteristics | G. Indicates blood accumulation in lungs |
| H. Signs of complications | H. Acute pulmonary edema is possible |
| I. Pulmonary function test | I. Indicates pulmonary status |

### III. Administer:
| A. O₂ therapy as ordered | A. Relieves dyspnea and tachypnea |
| B. Analgesic as ordered (usually morphine) | B. ↓ restlessness and dyspnea |

A. O$_2$ therapy as ordered — A. Relieves dyspnea and tachypnea

B. Analgesic as ordered (usually morphine) — B. ↓ restlessness and dyspnea

### IV. Perform/Provide:

A. Comfortable quiet environment — A. Strong emotions increase need for O$_2$

B. Semi-Fowler's position with pillows to support body — B. ↓ dyspnea, ↓ diaphragm, ↑ lung expansion

C. Anticipate patient's needs —place articles within easy reach — C. Limits O$_2$ demand

D. Deep breathing q 2 hr for 5–10 min — D. Expands lungs and prevents pneumonia

### V. Teach patient/family:

A. Need to avoid smokers, smoky environments — A. ↓ O$_2$ supply

B. Need to carry ID card with diagnosis, doctor's name and number, medications, dosage, and allergies — B. For emergency use if patient is unable to speak for self

C. Need to avoid persons with infections (URI) — C. ↑ chance of infection

D. Report to physician if persistent cough, shortness of breath, edema, or WT gain 5 lb — D. May indicate complication

E. About diagnostic test and procedures — E. Familiarity reduces anxiety which increases O$_2$ demand

F. Need for rest periods — F. ↓ O$_2$ demand

G. Avoid cold temperature (walk slowly, cover nose and mouth, dress warmly) — G. Causes vasoconstriction, increases BP, increases O$_2$ demand

---

**CONCEPT/NEED:** Transport/Circulation

**NURSING DIAGNOSIS:** Alteration in cardiac output: decreased related to venous pooling

**GOAL:** Increased cardiac output as evidenced by: stable BP, pulse, respirations during activity

**INTERVENTION**

**RATIONALE**

**I. Monitor, describe, record:**

A. Pulse rate and characteristics q 4 hr

B. BP q 4 hr

C. Heart sounds, pericardial friction rubs, ventricular gallop, and rales

A. Determines presence of impending arrhythmias, gather baseline data

B. Sign of left-sided heart failure

C. May indicate presence of arrhythmias

**II. Assess for:**

A. Cardiovascular status to include history, risk factors, and physical assessment

B. Chest x-ray

C. CVP above 12 cm $H_2O$

D. Increased circulation time. Beyond 15 sec arm to tongue, 8 sec arm to lungs

E. ECG

F. Lab studies to include BUN, creatinine, Hct, Hgb, SGOT, SGPT, LDH, bilirubin, albumin, PT, PTT, CPK

A. Needed for data base

B. Cardiac enlargement

C. Indicates decreased cardiac output

D. Increased due to venous pooling

E. May indicate ventricular hypertrophy/arrhythmias

F. Renal abnormalities and elevated enzymes confirm diagnosis

**III. Administer:**

A. Cardiac glycosides, nitrates, vasodilators as ordered

B. Sedatives as ordered

A. ↑ cardiac output, ↓ workload

B. ↓ agitation/cardiac workload

**IV. Perform/Provide:**

A. Antiembolic stockings as ordered. Reapply q 6 hr or PRN

A. Prevents emboli formation, ↑ venous return

| | |
|---|---|
| B. Comfortable, quiet environment | B. Agitation increases heart rate |
| C. Semi-Fowler's position | C. Prevents pooling of blood within pulmonary vessels |

## V. Teach patient/family:

| | |
|---|---|
| A. Need not to smoke | A. ↑ pulse, BP, and work of heart |
| B. Basic knowledge about disease process | B. ↓ anxiety |
| C. Diagnostic tests and procedures | C. ↓ anxiety |
| D. When and how to take medications and possible side effects | D. Insures safe administration |
| E. How to take pulse before administration of cardiac glycosides, symptoms of toxicity | E. ↓ chance of unsafe administration |
| F. Report to physician palpitations or chest pain | F. May indicate complications |

---

**CONCEPT/NEED:** Anxiety

**NURSING DIAGNOSIS:** Anxiety related to difficult breathing

**GOALS:** Reduction in anxiety as evidenced by: verbalization, pulse WNL, ability to sleep at night, ability to take slower deeper breaths

| **INTERVENTION** | **RATIONALE** |
|---|---|

### II. Assess for:

| | |
|---|---|
| A. Verbal and nonverbal clues to anxiety | A. May be unable to express feelings openly |
| B. Personal resources to cope with stress | B. Provides emotional support |
| C. Responses to information and treatments | C. May increase or decrease anxiety |
| D. Response to change in life style | D. Role conflict may occur due to illness |

E. Anxiety level of family (See Psychosocial Assessment for further guidelines, p. 31)

E. May upset patient

### III. Administer:
A. Sedatives and tranquilizers as ordered

A. ↓ tension, $O_2$ consumption

### IV. Perform/Provide:
A. Comfortable quiet environment

A. ↓ anxiety

B. Explanations about equipment, treatments

B. ↓ anxiety

C. Opportunity for expression of concerns, fears, and questions

C. Fosters open communication

D. Stay with patient during periods of crisis

D. Provides emotional support

E. Encourage participation in self-care as allowed by activity restrictions

E. Lessens sense of helplessness

F. Information about assistance from community agencies and support groups

F. Referral may be helpful for support

### V. Teach patient/family:
A. Avoid anxiety-producing situations

A. ↓ cardiac workload

B. About changes in patterns of living including work

B. Needed for compliance to reduce stress

C. Importance of communication with significant others

C. Provides for release of tension

---

**CONCEPT/NEED:** Mobility/Activity

**NURSING DIAGNOSIS:** Activity intolerance related to dyspnea

**GOALS:** Activity tolerance increased as evidenced by: regular rate/rhythm of respirations during activity; stable BP, pulse, during activity

| INTERVENTION | RATIONALE |
|---|---|
| **II. Assess for:** | |
| A. Amount of activity, self-care, interests, recreation, and usual sleep patterns | A. Provides baseline data |
| B. Paroxysmal nocturnal dyspnea | B. Indicates reduction in cardiac output |
| C. Patient's response to rest | C. Symptoms relieved or not relieved |
| **III. Administer:** | |
| A. Sedatives, tranquilizers or hypnotics as ordered | A. Provides rest, relieves insomnia |
| B. $O_2$ as ordered | B. Lack of $O_2$ causes restlessness |
| **IV. Perform/Provide:** | |
| A. Have call light and bedside table within easy reach | A. Limits fatigue |
| B. Comfortable quiet environment | B. Promotes rest |
| C. Avoid overtiring procedures, organize care to provide rest | C. ↓ fatigue |
| D. Back rubs, soft music, unhurried nursing care | D. Promotes relaxation |
| E. Encourage active or passive ROM | E. Prevents phlebitis, muscle wasting, and promotes circulation |
| F. Begin ambulation slowly dangling, then sitting in chair, then walking in room | F. Places less demand on heart |
| **V. Teach patient/family:** | |
| A. Balance rest and activity | A. Prevents fatigue |
| B. Avoid sitting in the same position over 2 hr | B. Avoids blood pooling in lower extremities |
| C. Avoid heavy lifting, pushing, and isometric exercise | C. Limits cardiac workload |
| D. Outline of activity permitted | D. ↑ compliance |

**CONCEPT/NEED:** Fluid/Electrolyte balance

**NURSING DIAGNOSIS:** Fluid volume excess related to edema

**GOAL:** Fluid retention will decrease as evidenced by: decreased pulmonary congestion on auscultation

| INTERVENTION | RATIONALE |
|---|---|
| **I. Monitor, describe, record:** | |
| A. I&O q 4–8 hr, and ratio | A. Indicates fluid buildup within system |
| B. WT at same time, in same clothing | B. May gain 10 lb before evidence of fluid retention |
| **II. Assess for:** | |
| A. Fluid and electrolyte status to include history, patterns, and present needs | A. Needed for data base |
| B. Laboratory values to include specific gravity, protein, creatinine, sodium | B. May indicate fluid retention |
| C. Estimate diaphoretic fluid loss | C. Sheets changed due to diaphoresis |
| D. Vomiting | D. Included in output |
| E. Degree of pitting edema (sacral and pedal) | E. Becomes obvious after 10 lb of retention |
| F. Lassitude, mental confusion, decreased urinary output from diuretics | F. Potassium loss |
| G. Muscle cramps, headaches, dizziness, skin rashes | G. Mineral depletion |
| **III. Administer:** | |
| A. Diuretics as ordered | A. ↑ fluid and sodium excretion |
| B. Potassium supplements as ordered | B. May be needed with potassium-depleting diuretics |
| **IV. Perform/Provide:** | |
| A. Semi-Fowler's position in bed or chair | A. ↓ edema |
| B. Move edematous extremities by supporting on palm | B. Fingertips may injure tissue |
| C. Low-sodium diet as ordered | C. Rids body of extracellular fluid retention |

## V. Teach patient/family:

A. Importance of daily WT, at same time, same clothing

A. Report any WT gain over 3 lb

B. Distribute ordered fluids over waking hr

B. ↓ thirst

C. Avoid foods that increase thirst if fluid is restricted

C. ↓ thirst

D. Use flavorings, spices, and herbs in place in salt, if low-sodium diet is ordered

D. Makes food more palatable

E. Rinse mouth well after using tooth cleansers and mouth-washes

E. Some contain large amounts of sodium

---

**CONCEPT/NEED:** Nutrition
Elimination

**NURSING DIAGNOSIS:** Potential alteration in nutrition: less than body requirements related to fatigue. Potential alteration in elimination: constipation related to immobility

**GOAL:** Nutrition will be maintained as evidenced by: eating small feedings 6/day, Hct and Hgb WNL. Bowel elimination will be maintained as evidenced by: BM pattern WNL for this patient

## INTERVENTION

## RATIONALE

### II. Assess for:

A. Nutrition and elimination status to include history, patterns, and present needs

A. Needed for data base

B. Nausea and vomiting

B. Affects appetite

### III. Administer:

A. Stool softeners as ordered

A. Prevents constipation

B. Oil retention enemas as ordered

B. Aids in defecation

C. Vitamin and mineral supplements as ordered

C. May be needed to insure proper vitamin/mineral

## IV. Perform/Provide:

A. Small frequent feedings (6/day)

A. Avoids excessive gastric filling, and abdominal distention which decreases lung capacity

B. Tempt appetite with food preferences that are allowed on diet

B. ↑ chance of eating proper diet

C. Low-calorie, low-residue, low-fat, nongas-forming foods as ordered

C. Includes diet restriction

D. Do not hurry patient with meals, open containers for patient

D. May take extended time, may need rest periods

E. Fluid and dietary adjustments to prevent constipation

E. Valsalva maneuver leads to increased strain on heart

## V. Teach patient/family:

A. Maintain prescribed diet

A. Needed to maintain health

B. Avoid very hot or very cold fluids

B. Not always an accepted belief

C. Serve 6 small feedings/day

C. ↓ lung capacity

D. Avoid caffeine drinks

D. ↑ heart rate

E. Avoid constipation and straining

E. Valsalva maneuver leads to increased strain on heart

# ■ Diminished Arterial Circulation to Extremities

**DEFINITION:** Reduced blood flow to peripheral tissues causing ischemia leading to possible infection, ulcer, or gangrene

**CONCEPT/NEED:** Transport/Circulation

**NURSING DIAGNOSIS:** Alteration in tissue perfusion related to reduced blood flow

**GOAL:** Increased tissue perfusion as evidenced by: pedal, popliteal pulses present and equal, decreased edema in extremities

| INTERVENTION | RATIONALE |
|---|---|
| **I. Monitor, describe, record:** | |
| A. Pedal and popliteal pulses QID | A. Decreased pulse is due to diminished circulation |
| B. Pulse q 4 hr | B. Indicates circulation |
| **II. Assess for:** | |
| A. Hair loss, pigmentation, rashes, and decrease in temperature of extremities. Also, cellulitis, necrosis, gangrene, edema | A. Diminished blood supply decreases $O_2$ to cells |
| B. Loss of sensation or numbness in extremities | B. Related to decreased blood supply |
| C. Thickened nails | C. Accumulation of cornified material due to lack of $O_2$ |
| D. Pallor of extremities | D. ↑ with elevation, ↓ when not elevated |
| E. Elevated plasma lipids | E. ↑ with disorder |
| F. Results of arteriogram, thermography, plethysmography (See Cardiovascular Assessment, p. 59) | F. To assess narrowing of arterial lumen, temperature loss in extremities. Change in size of extremity due to altered blood supply |

### III. Administer:
A. Anticoagulants as ordered

A. Prevents formation of thrombi or emboli

B. Vasodilators as ordered

B. ↑ arterial lumen size

C. Antilipidemics if ordered

C. ↓ lipid levels

### IV. Perform/Provide:
A. Low-cholesterol, low-calorie diet as ordered

A. Helps halt lipid accumulation in arterial lumen

B. Environmental temp at 21°C (70°F). Use added clothing to keep warm if needed

B. Limits vasoconstriction

C. Adequate fluids

C. ↓ viscosity

### V. Teach patient/family:
A. Basic knowledge about disease and treatments

A. Familiarity reduces anxiety

B. Not to remain in one position too long

B. ↓ venous stasis

C. Avoid crossing legs and sit with a distance of 2 fingers between chair and popliteal space

C. Prevents arterial compression

D. Drink adequate fluids

D. ↓ viscosity of blood

E. Avoid exposure to cold or excessive heat

E. Limits vasoconstriction

F. Avoid tight-fitting or constrictive clothing (garters)

F. ↓ circulation

G. Sleep with head of bed elevated (6 in)

G. ↑ arterial blood flow to extremities

H. Avoid smoking

H. Nicotine is a vasoconstrictor

I. Name of medications, dosage, time, purpose, and side effects

I. Insures safe administration

J. Avoid OTC drugs

J. May interact with prescribed meds

K. Watch for bleeding gums, hematuria, easy bruisability, blood in stools

K. Effects from anticoagulant therapy

---

**CONCEPT/NEED:** Pain

**NURSING DIAGNOSIS:** Alteration in comfort: pain related to reduced blood flow in extremities

**GOAL:** Increased comfort as evidenced by: verbalization, asking for less pain medication, no grimacing, pulse WNL

## INTERVENTION

## RATIONALE

II. **Assess for:**
   A. Pain—sharp, vise-like occurring in foot, calf, buttocks. Increased with elevation of legs
   B. Intermittent claudication

   C. How pain is relieved

   D. Usual sleep patterns
   E. Edema

A. ↑ with poor circulation in extremities

B. Pain which increases with activity relieved by rest
C. Needed to treat pain conservatively
D. Needed for data base
E. Indicates fluid retention

III. **Administer:**
   A. Analgesics as ordered

A. For control of pain

IV. **Perform/Provide:**
   A. Reposition extremities q 2 hr
   B. Alternate undisturbed rest and activity
   C. Use bed cradle

A. Relieves pressure
B. Prevents overtiring

C. Keeps cover off affected area

V. **Teach patient/family**
   A. Alternate undisturbed rest and activity
   B. Walk until pain develops, stand still to decrease pain before continuing

A. ↑ comfort

B. Promotes development of collateral circulation

---

**CONCEPT/NEED:** Skin integrity

**NURSING DIAGNOSIS:** Impairment of skin integrity related to poor tissue perfusion

**GOAL:** Skin integrity maintained as evidenced by: absence of breaks in skin, ulcer, skin atrophy, absence of delayed healing

| INTERVENTION | RATIONALE |
|---|---|
| **II. Assess for:** | |
| A. Thickening, drying, cracking areas of ulceration on skin QD | A. ↓ blood supply, ↑ tissue breakdown |
| B. Temperature q 4 hr | B. Sign of infection |
| **IV. Perform/Provide:** | |
| A. Bed cradle over affected area, foot boards, and padding | A. Helps prevent skin breakdown |
| B. Use heel guards or white cotton socks, lambswool between toes | B. Protects pressure points |
| C. Turn q 2 hr while on bedrest | C. Prevents decubitus ulcer formation |
| D. Assist patient out of bed | D. Prevents falls |
| E. Hygiene, use small amount of mild soap, rinse well, dry gently, avoid rubbing | E. Soap dries skin |
| F. Apply lotion | F. Prevents cracking |
| G. Avoid adhesive tape | G. Chance of tissue injury |
| H. Cut toenails straight across | H. Prevents injury to tissues around nail |
| I. Leave light on at night | I. Prevents falls which may cause tissue damage |
| **V. Teach patient/family:** | |
| A. Inspect for injury and pressure areas | A. ↓ chance of complication |
| B. Wear only properly fitting socks and shoes | B. ↓ constriction |
| C. Notify physician of skin breaks that do not heal in 2–3 days or become infected | C. Potential for further breakdown or infection |
| D. Not to cut, file nails, or use OTC medications on corns or calluses | D. Care should be given by a podiatrist |

E. Turn on lights when getting up at night

E. Prevents falls

F. Not to apply heat directly to legs (hot water bottle or heating pad may help)

F. Burns may lead to tissue breakdown

G. Clean small cuts or abrasions with soap and water

G. Prevents infection

# ■ Hypertension

**DEFINITION:** The sustained elevation of blood pressure above 140 mm Hg systolic and 90 mm Hg diastolic or a sustained elevation above an individual's norms leading to hypertensive heart disease

**CONCEPT/NEED:** Transport/Circulation

**NURSING DIAGNOSIS:** Alteration in tissue perfusion related to increased BP

**GOAL:** Adequate tissue perfusion as evidenced by: BP WNL, absence of signs or symptoms of complications in cardiovascular system

## INTERVENTION

I. **Monitor, describe, record:**
   A. Pulse rate and characteristics q 4 hr (tachycardia, bradycardia)
   B. Apical/radial pulse BID
   C. Peripheral pulses QD

   D. BP q 4 hr, both arms, sitting and standing

   E. Narrowed pulse pressure
   F. Cardiac arrhythmias

II. **Assess for:**
   A. Orthostatic hypotension to include pallor, faintness
   B. Distended neck veins or epistaxis
   C. Changes in respiration and airway patency q 4 hr
   D. ECG and x-ray results (See Cardiovascular Assessment, p. 59)

## RATIONALE

A. Indicates cardiac status

B. Indicates pulse deficit
C. Diminished femoral pulse suggests coarctation of the aorta
D. Difference of over 10 mm suggests arterial compression or obstruction
E. Indicates reduced circulation
F. Indicates angina or MI

A. Indicates changes in blood flow

B. Sign of hypertensive heart failure

C. Identifies complications

D. Reveal abnormalities (narrowing of coronary vessels), hypertrophy of heart

### III. Administer:
A. Antihypertensive medications as ordered and observe for side effects

A. ↓ peripheral resistance and suppress renin production

### IV. Perform/Provide:
A. Restful environment

A. Limits emotions that increase arterial pressure

B. Position of comfort when in bed

B. ↓ pain in area

C. Assistance in getting out of bed slowly

C. Prevents orthostatic hypotension

### V. Teach patient/family:
A. Take BP and pulse and keep record

A. Variations can be observed with regular record

B. The nature and complications of disease

B. May reduce fear or assist with identifying complications

C. Purpose of tests and diagnostic procedures

C. ↓ anxiety

D. Avoid excessive heat and alcohol

D. Causes vasodilation resulting in fainting by potentiating drugs

E. Avoid standing in one place for extended periods of time

E. Vessels in legs relax allowing pooling of blood which causes faintness

F. Caution when driving or operating machinery

F. Drowsiness is side effect of drug

G. Not to take more or less of drug than prescribed

G. Accurate administration prevents toxicity or undermedication

H. Not to D/C drug suddenly

H. May increase BP quickly

I. Report any symptoms to physician

I. May need to adjust medications

J. Avoid OTC drugs

J. May interact with prescribed drugs

K. Side effects of prescribed drugs

K. ↓ tension

---

**CONCEPT/NEED:** Nutrition
Fluid/Electrolyte balance

**NURSING DIAGNOSIS:** Alteration in nutrition: more than body requirements related to inappropriate intake. Fluid volume excess related to edema

**GOAL:** Adequate nutrition as evidenced by: following dietary restrictions. Adequate fluid volume as evidenced by: lack of edema

## INTERVENTION

I. **Monitor, describe, record:**
   A. Height, WT QD at same time, scale, and clothing
   B. I&O q 8 hr if needed

II. **Assess for:**
   A. Nutrition, fluid, electrolyte, and elimination status to include history, patterns, present needs
   B. Aldosterone, protein, creatinine, 17-keto-steroid results
   C. Edema of lower extremities
   D. Nausea and vomiting
   E. Potassium levels
   F. WT changes

III. **Administer:**
   A. Potassium as ordered

   B. Diuretics as ordered

IV. **Perform/Provide:**
   A. Low calories, cholesterol, low sodium as ordered for diet

   B. Fluid intake as determined by individual need

V. **Teach patient/family:**
   A. Dietary restrictions of calories, salt, and animal fat

## RATIONALE

A. Detects sudden WT change caused by fluid retention or loss
B. Detects water retention causing an increased blood volume and higher BP

A. Detects early symptoms of hypertension

B. Test of renal function

C. Indicates fluid retention
D. Indicates fluid loss
E. Diuretics deplete potassium level
F. Rauwolfia drugs increase appetite and cause WT gain

A. Replace potassium loss resulting from enuresis
B. ↓ circulating blood volume, ↓ cardiac output

A. Eliminates overweight, to reduce workload of heart, prevents edema

B. Maintains hydration

A. ↓ sodium and blood volume, ↓ heart workload

B. Avoid eating or drinking large amounts

B. ↑ heart rate

C. Limitation on tea, coffee, and alcohol

C. ↑ heart rate

D. Importance of continuing medications prescribed and reporting side effects

D. Need to reduce BP with lowest dose causing least side effects

E. Importance of maintaining appropriate WT

E. Overweight increases workload of heart

---

**CONCEPT/NEED:** Anxiety

**NURSING DIAGNOSIS:** Anxiety related to inability to perform role in family.

**GOAL:** Reduction of anxiety as evidenced by: verbalization, developing plan for life style changes, pulse WNL

## INTERVENTION

## RATIONALE

II. **Assess for:**
   A. Verbal and nonverbal clues to anxiety

   A. May be unable to express feelings openly

   B. Personal resources to cope with stress

   B. Provides persons to assist in giving emotional support

   C. Responses to information and treatments

   C. May increase or decrease anxiety

   D. Response to change in life style

   D. Role conflict may occur due to illness

   E. Anxiety level of family (See Psychosocial Assessment for further guidelines, p. 31)

   E. May upset patient

III. **Administer:**
   A. Sedatives and tranquilizers as ordered

   A. ↓ tension, indirectly BP

## IV. Perform/Provide:

A. Comfortable quiet environment
A. ↓ anxiety

B. Explanations about equipment, treatment
B. ↓ anxiety

C. Opportunity for expression of concerns, fears, and questions
C. Fosters open communication

D. Stay with patient during periods of crisis
D. Provides emotional support

E. Encourage participation in self-care as allowed by activity restrictions
E. ↓ sense of helplessness

F. Information about assistance from community agencies and support groups
F. Provides emotional support

## V. Teach patient/family:

A. Avoid anxiety-producing situations
A. ↓ cardiac workload

B. About changes in patterns of living including work
B. Helps planning for future

C. Importance of communication with significant others
C. Provides for release of tension

D. Not to D/C drug no matter how well he or she feels
D. A lifelong illness

---

**CONCEPT/NEED:** Mobility/Activity

**NURSING DIAGNOSIS:** Activity intolerance related to fatigue

**GOALS:** Activity maintained as evidenced by: adherence to daily exercise program without fatigue, BP and pulse WNL after activity

### INTERVENTION

### RATIONALE

## II. Assess for:

A. Amount of activity, self-care, interests, recreation
A. Provides baseline data

## IV. Perform/Provide:
A. Encourage active or passive ROM. Progressive ambulation regimen. Ambulation as tolerated

A. Promotes circulation

B. Support and/or assist in self-care

B. Prevents injury

## V. Teach patient/family:
A. Program for regular exercises/rest (especially walking)

A. ↓ tension

B. Avoid fatigue

B. Stresses heart

C. Engage in activities that do not produce stress

C. ↓ stress, ↓ heart rate

D. Outline of activity permitted

D. Prevents overexertion

E. Monitoring WT. May decrease BP and cardiac workload

E. May never need medications

# ■ Myocardial Infarction

**DEFINITION:** The destruction or necrosis of an area of the myocardium resulting from a decrease or cessation of blood flow caused by a thrombus or atherosclerosis in a coronary artery

**CONCEPT/NEED:** Transport/Circulation

**NURSING DIAGNOSIS:** Alteration in tissue perfusion related to reduced blood supply

**GOAL:** Tissue perfusion will be maintained as evidenced by: warm extremities, equal, strong peripheral pulses

| INTERVENTION | RATIONALE |
|---|---|
| **I. Monitor, describe, record:** | |
| A. Pulse, respirations, and characteristics q 4 hr | A. VS indicate increased anxiety which increases work on heart |
| B. Apical/radial pulse BID | B. Arrhythmia detection |
| C. Peripheral pulses | C. Indicates peripheral circulation |
| D. BP q 4 hr lying and standing both arms | D. Indicates tissue perfusion in both arms |
| E. ECG | E. May lead to arrhythmias |
| F. Heart sound S1 and S2, murmur, gallup, pericardial rub | F. Indicates valvular defects (CHF, post-MI complications) |
| **II. Assess for:** | |
| A. S&S of complications | A. Heart failure, cardiogenic shock |
| B. Cardiac enzymes (SGOT, CPK, LDH), creatinine, ESR, WBC | B. Indicates cardiac function |
| C. ECG and x-ray results (See Cardiovascular Assessment, p. 59) | C. Reveals abnormalities such as narrowing of coronary vessels or heart enlargement |

## III. Administer:

A. Anticoagulants as ordered — A. Prevents intravascular clots

B. Beta-adrenergic blocking agents or calcium blockers as ordered — B. ↓ O₂ requirement of myocardium

C. Vasodilators and observe for side effects and response — C. Dilates coronary vessels increasing blood flow to myocardium

D. Antiarrhythmics as ordered — D. Regulate conduction and rhythm

## IV. Perform/Provide:

A. Bedrest complete or as ordered — A. ↓ stress on heart

B. Comfortable, quiet environment — B. Strong emotions increase heart's workload

C. Position of comfort — C. Prevents excessive pooling within pulmonary vessels

## V. Teach patient/family:

A. Need not to smoke — A. ↑ pulse, BP, and work of the heart

B. Disease process and treatment — B. Helps prevent recurrence

C. Restrictions in activity — C. Heavy exertion increases work of heart, prevents healing

D. When and how to take medications and possible side effects — D. Insures safe administration

E. About diagnostic tests and procedures — E. Familiarity reduces anxiety

F. How to take pulse measurements before administration of cardiotonics — F. Do not administer if pulse is below 60 bpm

---

**CONCEPT/NEED:** Pain

**NURSING DIAGNOSIS:** Alteration in comfort: pain related to decreased blood supply to myocardium

**GOAL:** Increased comfort as evidenced by: verbalization, no grimacing, pulse WNL, decreasing use of analgesics

| **INTERVENTION** | **RATIONALE** |
|---|---|

**II. Assess for:**

A. Characteristics of pain, crushing, stabbing or heavy weight. Radiating to left shoulder, arm down to wrist and fingers or to neck and jaw. Duration of 5 min or longer

   A. Complete stoppage of blood supply to myocardium

B. Associated symptoms of dyspnea, pallor, sweating, dizziness, faintness

   B. Complete stoppage of blood supply with these associated symptoms

C. Pain is unrelieved by rest or nitroglycerin

   C. Angina is relieved by rest or nitroglycerin

**III. Administer:**

A. Narcotic analgesics as ordered

   A. ↓ pain

B. O₂ therapy as ordered

   B. ↓ pain, ↑ O₂

**IV. Perform/Provide:**

A. Stay with patient during periods of pain

   A. Reassurance reduces anxiety and cardiac workload

B. Position of comfort

   B. Helps to control pain

C. Comfortable, quiet environment

   C. Limiting stimuli will decrease anxiety

**V. Teach patient/family:**

A. Importance of calling physician if pain continues longer than 20 min after taking vasodilators

   A. May indicate MI rather than angina

---

**CONCEPT/NEED:** Anxiety

**NURSING DIAGNOSIS:** Anxiety related to possible death

**GOAL:** Decreased anxiety as evidenced by: verbalization, warm hands, ability to sleep at night

| INTERVENTION | RATIONALE |
|---|---|
| **II. Assess for:** | |
| A. Verbal and nonverbal clues of anxiety | A. Patient may be unable to openly communicate. Open communication reduces stress |
| B. Personal resources to cope with stress | B. Provides emotional support |
| C. Responses to information and treatments | C. Treatments and information may increase or decrease anxiety |
| D. Changes in life style (See Psychosocial Assessment for further guidelines, p. 31) | D. Role conflict may occur due to illness |
| **IV. Perform/Provide:** | |
| A. Accepting environment to state feelings | A. Provides emotional support |
| B. Environment that avoids anxiety-producing situations | B. ↓ anxiety |
| C. Referral for counseling for extremely anxious individual | C. May need professional psychiatric intervention |
| D. Encouragement to perform self-care as able | D. ↓ sense of helplessness and emotional trauma |
| **V. Teach patient/family:** | |
| A. Avoid anxiety-producing situations | A. May lead to increased workload of heart |
| B. Possible changes in patterns of living to include work if needed | B. Changes may be needed to reduce anxiety |
| C. Importance of need to deal with fears regarding role change and sexual ability | C. Open communication lessens fear of unknown |

---

**CONCEPT/NEED:** Lifestyle

**NURSING DIAGNOSIS:** Ineffective individual coping related to identifiable stressors

**GOAL:** Ineffective individual coping will be minimized as evidenced by: discussing how life style will need to be altered, verbalization and follow through with decision to alter life style as needed

| INTERVENTION | RATIONALE |
|---|---|
| **I. Monitor, describe, record:** | |
|   A. Usual methods of coping with stress | A. Identifies coping patterns |
| **II. Assess for:** | |
|   A. Stress level past and present | A. History is needed for data |
|   B. How patient views this illness and amount of life disruption | B. Indicates importance of changes that will need to be made |
|     (See Work, Play Assessments, p. 36) | |
| **III. Administer:** | |
|   A. Antianxiety medications as ordered | A. ↓ stress on heart |
|   B. Hypnotics as ordered | B. To provide rest |
| **V. Teach patient/family:** | |
|   A. Relaxation techniques | A. Provide rest for adequate life planning |
|   B. Process for problem solving | B. Aids in dealing with patient's problems |

# ■ Thrombophlebitis/Venous Thrombosis

**DEFINITION:** An inflammation of the vein wall with clot formation. Usually occurs in veins of the lower extremities as a result of reduced blood flow. Clot formation without inflammation is called phlebothrombosis

**CONCEPT/NEED:** Transport/Circulation

**NURSING DIAGNOSIS:** Alteration in tissue perfusion related to obstruction

**GOAL:** Adequate tissue perfusion as evidenced by: equal, strong pedal, popliteal pulses, skin—warm, dry on extremities

| INTERVENTION | RATIONALE |
|---|---|
| **I. Monitor, describe, record:** | |
| A. Pulse, respirations, and characteristics q 4 hr | A. Indicates cardiac status |
| B. Apical/radial pulse BID | B. Arrhythmia detection |
| C. Peripheral pulses | C. Peripheral blood flow |
| D. BP q 4 hr lying and standing both arms | D. Indicates pulse deficit |
| E. Size of affected extremities q 4 hr | E. Can occur with edema |
| **II. Assess for:** | |
| A. History, risk factors, life style with cardiovascular status (See Cardiovascular Assessment, p. 59) | A. Needed for data base |
| B. S&S of complications | B. Common complication is pulmonary embolism |
| C. Results of PTT, PT, Lee White, radioactive iodine study | C. Indicates anticoagulant therapy adequacy |

Venous pressure

Reveals pressure in occluded saphenous vein

Ultrasonic Doppler flow
Plethysmography

Reveals decrease in blood flow
Reveals change in limb size due to circulation

## III. Administer:

| | |
|---|---|
| A. Anticoagulants as ordered | A. Prevents intravascular clots |
| B. Fibrinolytic agents as ordered | B. Enhances dissolution of clot |
| C. Vasodilators and observe for side effects and response | C. Dilates coronary vessels increasing blood flow to aid in absorption of clots |
| D. Whole blood or vitamin K as ordered | D. If bleeding occurs because of anticoagulant therapy |

## IV. Perform/Provide:

| | |
|---|---|
| A. Bedrest complete or as ordered | A. ↓ chance of clot being dislodged |
| B. Elevation of extremity as ordered | B. ↓ venous congestion and edema |
| C. Hot wet dressings or heat cradle | C. Promotes circulation |

## V. Teach patient/family:

| | |
|---|---|
| A. Not to rub or massage affected leg | A. Danger of releasing clot to lung |
| B. Wear elastic stockings as ordered | B. Minimizes venous pressure |
| C. Avoid tight constrictive clothing and long periods of standing | C. May reduce circulation |
| D. Need to carry ID card with doctor's name, diagnosis, medications, and allergies | D. For emergency use |
| E. Watch for bleeding gums, hematuria, bruisability, blood in stools | E. Effects from anticoagulant therapy |
| F. Elevate legs during convalescent period | F. ↓ venous pooling, ↑ venous return |
| G. Use electric razor for shaving | G. Prevents bleeding from cuts |

**CONCEPT/NEED:** Comfort

**NURSING DIAGNOSIS:** Alteration in comfort: pain related to inflammation

**GOAL:** Increased comfort as evidenced by: absence of pain, warmth in extremities, verbalization

| INTERVENTION | RATIONALE |
|---|---|
| **II. Assess for:** | |
| A. Characteristics of pain | A. Swelling and edema increase pain |
| B. Positive Homan's sign | B. Pain in leg on forced dorsiflexion of the foot |
| C. Temperature, color of affected limb | C. Redness, warmth, signs of inflammatory process |
| D. Skin breakdown under elastic hose | D. Inflammation may occur due to constriction which reduces blood flow |
| **III. Administer:** | |
| A. Analgesics as ordered | A. ↓ pain |
| **IV. Perform/Provide:** | |
| A. Backrubs, warm drinks, unhurried nursing care | A. ↑ comfort |
| B. Position as ordered, change position to relieve pressure | B. Prevents skin breakdown |
| C. Apply heat or cold as ordered | C. ↓ inflammation |
| D. Involve in diversional activities | D. Releases tension |
| E. Move extremities by supporting with palms | E. Fingertips may injure tissues |
| **V. Teach patient/family:** | |
| A. Reduce WT as ordered, avoid prolonged standing, crossing legs, and constrictive clothing. Elevate legs as ordered | A. Improves venous return |

**CONCEPT/NEED:** Sleep
Activity/Mobility

**NURSING DIAGNOSIS:** Potential sleep pattern disturbance related to pain. Activity intolerance related to pain

**GOAL:** Adequate sleep as evidenced by: sleeping 6–8 hr/night. Activity tolerance as evidenced by: participation in progressive exercise program

## INTERVENTION

**II. Assess for:**
   A. Amount of acitivity, self-care, interests, recreation, and usual sleep patterns

**IV. Perform/Provide:**
   A. Bedrest during acute state
   B. Exercise program once threat of embolus is over. Ambulate 5–10 min q 1 hr
   C. Active or passive ROM to unaffected extremities
   D. Alternate ambulation with bedrest

**V. Teach patient/family:**
   A. Increase walking distance slowly until 1–2 miles/day
   B. Alternate activity and rest periods with legs elevated
   C. Elevate head of bed 6–8 in

## RATIONALE

A. Needed for data base

A. Prevents embolus
B. Promotes circulation

C. ↑ circulation, ↓ muscle wasting

D. ↓ pooling of blood

A. ↑ circulation, ↓ chance of subsequent clot formation
B. ↓ venous pooling

C. ↓ venous pooling, ↑ venous return

# ■ Varicose Veins/Venous Insufficiency

**DEFINITION:** Varicose veins are lengthened and dilated superficial veins resulting from incompetent valves in surface veins commonly found in the lower extremities. Venous insufficiency is a condition resulting from venous valve incompetence in legs caused by consistent high venous pressure

**CONCEPT/NEED:** Transport/Circulation

**NURSING DIAGNOSIS:** Alteration in tissue perfusion: decreased related to obstruction

**GOAL:** Adequate cardiac output as evidenced by: equal, strong, pedal, popliteal pulses, lack of leg edema

## INTERVENTION

I. **Monitor, describe, record:**
   A. Pulse and characteristics q 4 hr
   B. BP q 4 hr
   C. Peripheral pulses, inguinal pulses, color, temperature q 6 hr

II. **Assess for:**
   A. Walking test

   B. Trendelenburg test

   C. Venography

   D. Complications such as leg edema, hemorrhage

## RATIONALE

A. Indicates cardiac status

B. Indicates cardiac status

C. Indicates peripheral blood flow

A. ↑ venous pressure during walking with rapid return when walking stops (normal functioning)

B. Will fill from above rather than below an applied tourniquet

C. Reveals abnormalities in sharp and valvular cusps

D. Edema from superficial thrombosis, hemorrhage from increased pressure, weak vein wall

### III. Administer:
A. Solution of sclerosing drugs
A. Induces vein fibrosis
B. Semirigid paste boot as ordered
B. Stabilizes ulcer and heals

### IV. Perform/Provide:
A. Elevation of extremity as ordered. Prevention of long periods of standing. Elevate foot of bed 6–8 in
A. ↓ venous pooling, ↑ venous return
B. Elastic stockings as ordered
B. Edema is minimized

### V. Teach patient/family:
A. Care of paste boot if applied
A. Ensures patient compliance
B. Wear elastic stockings as ordered
B. Minimizes venous pressure
C. Avoid tight constrictive clothing and long periods of standing
C. May reduce circulation
D. Elevate legs during convalescent period
D. ↓ venous pooling, ↑ venous return

---

**CONCEPT/NEED:** Pain

**NURSING DIAGNOSIS:** Alteration in comfort: pain related to obstruction

**GOAL:** Increased comfort as evidenced by: absence of pain, warmth in extremities, verbalization

## INTERVENTION

### II. Assess for:
A. Characteristics of pain
B. Positive Homan's sign
C. Temperature, color of affected limb
D. Skin breakdown under elastic hose

### III. Administer:
A. Analgesics as ordered

## RATIONALE

A. Swelling and edema increase pain
B. Indicates thrombosis
C. Redness, warmth, signs of inflammatory process
D. Inflammation may occur


A. ↓ pain

## IV. Perform/Provide:

| | |
|---|---|
| A. Backrubs, warm drinks, un-hurried nursing care | A. ↑ comfort |
| B. Position as ordered, change position to relieve pressure | B. Prevents skin breakdown |
| C. Apply heat or cold as or-dered | C. ↓ inflammation/perfusion |
| D. Involve in diversional activ-ities | D. Releases tension |
| E. Move extremities by sup-porting with palms | E. Fingertips may injure tissues |

## V. Teach patient/family:

| | |
|---|---|
| A. Reduce WT as ordered, avoid prolonged standing, crossing legs, and constric-tive clothing. Elevate legs as ordered | A. Controls symptoms |

---

**CONCEPT/NEED:** Safety

**NURSING DIAGNOSIS:** Potential for injury related to improper foot care

**GOAL:** Absence of injury as evidenced by: smooth, clean feet, legs, seek-ing a podiatrist for problems with foot care

## INTERVENTION

## RATIONALE

### II. Assess for:

| | |
|---|---|
| A. Complications hemorrhage, thrombophlebitis, ulcer for-mation, and symptoms of emboli, allergic reaction to sclerosing drugs | A. Identifies complications |
| B. Skin breakdown under elas-tic hose q 6 hr | B. May go unnoticed |

### V. Teach patient/family:

| | |
|---|---|
| A. Care of leg ulcers | A. Prevents infection |
| B. Remove elastic stockings BID | B. Assesses for skin breakdown |
| C. Keep legs warm and dry | C. Promotes circulation |

# ■ Vein Ligation/Stripping

**DEFINITION:** Ligation of the saphenous vein at the groin and the stripping of the full length of the saphenous vein from groin to ankle. Additional incisions may be made into veins to remove varicosities

**CONCEPT/NEED:** Transport/Circulation

**NURSING DIAGNOSIS:** Alteration in tissue perfusion: decreased related to trauma

**GOAL:** Adequate cardiac output as evidenced by: normal skin color, peripheral pulses equal, strong

| INTERVENTION | RATIONALE |
|---|---|
| **I. Monitor, describe, record:** | |
| A. Pulse and characteristics q 4 hr | A. Indicates cardiac status |
| B. BP q 4 hr | B. Indicates cardiac status |
| C. Peripheral pulses, inguinal pulses, color, temperature q 6 hr (See Pre-Operative, Post-Operative Assessment, p. 13, p. 17) | C. Indicates peripheral blood flow |
| **II. Assess for:** | |
| A. Walking test | A. ↑ venous pressure during walking with rapid return when walking stops (normal functioning) |
| B. Trendelenburg test | B. Will fill from above rather than below an applied tourniquet |
| C. Venography | C. Reveals abnormalities in sharp and valvular cusps |
| D. Complications such as leg edema, hemorrhage | D. Edema from superficial thrombosis, hemorrhage from increased pressure, weak vein wall |

## IV. Perform/Provide:

A. Elevation of extremity as ordered. Prevention of long periods of standing. Elevate foot of bed 6–8 in

A. ↓ venous pooling, ↑ venous return

B. Elastic stockings as ordered

B. Edema is minimized

## V. Teach patient/family:

A. Care of paste boot if applied

A. Insures patient compliance

B. Wear elastic stockings as ordered

B. Minimizes venous pressure

C. Avoid tight constrictive clothing and long periods of standing

C. May reduce circulation

D. Elevate legs during convalescent period

D. ↓ venous pooling, ↑ venous return

---

**CONCEPT/NEED:** Pain
Activity/Immobility

**NURSING DIAGNOSIS:** Alteration in comfort: pain related to incision. Potential activity intolerance related to pain

**GOAL:** Increased comfort as evidenced by: verbalization, decreased use of analgesics. Activity tolerance as evidenced by ambulation within 24 hr, increasing ambulation without use of analgesics

## INTERVENTION

## RATIONALE

### II. Assess for:

A. Characteristics of pain, cramping, numbness

A. Needed for data base

B. Amount of activity self-care, recreation, interests, usual sleep patterns

B. Needed for data base

### III. Administer:

A. Analgesics as ordered

A. ↓ pain

## IV. Perform/Provide:

A. Assist with ambulation within 24 hr. Perform active and passive ROM to unaffected extremities q 4 hr. Gradually lengthen walking periods

A. Promotes circulation

B. Elevate foot of bed 6–8 in

B. Prevents venous pooling

## V. Teach patient/family:

A. Reduce WT as ordered, avoid prolonged standing, crossing legs, and constrictive clothing. Elevate legs as ordered

A. Controls symptoms

B. Walk 5 min q 1 hr and progress to 1 40 min walk QD

B. Promotes circulation gradually

# RESPIRATORY SYSTEM STANDARDS

- Respiratory System Assessment
- Atelectasis
- Bronchitis/Bronchiectasis/Asthma
- Chronic Obstructive Pulmonary Disease
- Fractured Ribs
- Pleurisy/Pleuritis/Pleural Effusion
- Pneumonia
- Pneumothorax/Hemothorax
- Pulmonary Edema
- Pulmonary Tumors
- Tracheostomy

# ■ Respiratory System Assessment

**DEFINITION:** The collection of a data base concerning the respiratory system and its functional capabilities to be used in identifying nursing problems related to oxygenation

**CONCEPT/NEED:** Oxygenation

## I. Interview for and record past history:
A. Previous lung or chest conditions such as asthma, TB, COPD
B. Family members with lung or chest conditions
C. Previous operations, injuries, or chronic medical conditions related to lungs
D. Allergies, immunizations
E. Smoking/day and number of years
F. Exposure to environmental pollution, occupational
G. URI and frequency
H. Cough and characteristics, sneezing
I. Shortness of breath, wheezing and how remedied
J. Position for sleeping (pillows used)
K. Pain in chest
L. Dizziness, chills, fever, edema, confusion
M. Usual respiratory rate/min and factors that increase rate of cause difficulty
N. Customary medications taken for cough, URI and response (prescribed and OTC)
O. Past chest x-rays, PPD, pulmonary function studies or other tests and results

## II. Interview for and record present history:
A. Chief complaint
B. Onset and length of illness
C. Knowledge of disease, procedures, and planned therapy
D. Results of Hct, Hgb, electrolytes, ESR, ABGs, pulmonary function studies, chest x-ray, ECG, lung scan, sputum
E. AP to lateral diameter between 1:2, 5:7
F. Ribs slope at 45 degree angle downward
G. Symmetry in shape, movement, and expansion of chest
H. Symmetry of clavicles and scapulae
I. Deviations of spinal column (kyphosis, scoliosis)

J. Use of diaphragm, chest, or abdominal movement in breathing
K. Position for optimal breathing
L. Skin lesions, irritations
M. Color of skin, lips, nails, ears (pallor, cyanosis)
N. Chest hair
O. Capillary refill of nailbeds
P. Clubbing of fingers
Q. Flaring nostrils, mouth breathing
R. Confusion, restlessness
S. Cough, frequency, productive, nonproductive
T. Sputum color, amount, odor, consistency

## IV. Palpation for:
A. Skin warm, dry, smooth to touch
B. Pain, tenderness or masses in chest
C. Muscles, intercostal spaces firm, smooth
D. Bulging or retraction of interspaces during respirations
E. Retraction of suprasternal or substernal areas during respirations
F. Trachea in midline
G. Pulsations at suprasternal notch
H. Anterior and posterior chest wall expansion and symmetry
I. Vocal or tactile fremitus and whether increased or decreased and location

## V. Percussion for:
A. Resonance over lung fields, anterior and posterior (loud intensity, low pitch, long duration, a hollow sound)
B. Hyperresonance in overinflated lungs (loud intensity, deep pitch, prolonged duration, more hollow sound)
C. Tympany in areas of air enclosed in sac (high pitch, drum-like)
D. Dull sound over solid area such as liver, heart, scapulae, vertebrae (medium intensity, pitch, duration)
E. Flatness over solid or fluid mass (soft intensity, high pitch, short duration)
F. Assess for bilateral comparison results

## VI. Auscultation for:
A. Same voice sound intensity bilaterally
B. Louder sounds near airways and decreasing at periphery
C. Whispers faint and indistinct
D. Adventitious sound
   1. Pleural friction rub (grating, leathery)
   2. Rales (coarse, fine, bubbling, crackling)

      3. Rhonchi (low, rumbling, bubbling)
      4. Wheezes (high pitched, whistling)
      5. Stridor (wheezing on inspiration)
E.  Breath sounds
      1. Bronchovesicular over airways (upper 1/3 of sternum) are medium to high pitch, moderate loudness and have blowing muffled sound
      2. Vesicular over rest of lung fields (mainly periphery) are medium to low pitch, low amplitude, breezy, swishing
      3. Tracheal over trachea are loud, high pitched, tubular, harsh
      4. Bronchial over manubrium are high pitched, loud, tubular, harsh
      5. Assess for decreased or absent breath sounds in same areas
      6. Assess as abnormal if any of these breath sounds are found in any other area of lung fields other than where expected

# ■ Atelectasis

**DEFINITION:** The collapse of lung tissue resulting from a mucus plug or secretions in the bronchi preventing the passage of air to and from the alveoli

**CONCEPT/NEED:** Oxygenation

**NURSING DIAGNOSIS:** Ineffective breathing pattern related to obstruction

**GOAL:** Effective breathing pattern as evidenced by: deep, clear breath sounds upon auscultation

| INTERVENTION | RATIONALE |
|---|---|
| **I. Monitor, describe, record:** | |
| A. Breath sounds q 2–4 hr. Respiration rate and quality | A. Diminished or absent over affected area |
| B. B/P, apical pulse q 4 hr | B. BP change in hypoxia. First increased, then decreased |
| **II. Assess for:** | |
| A. Shortness of breath, cyanosis, restlessness (See Respiratory Assessment, p. 105) | A. ↓ O₂ supply |
| B. Egophony with auscultation | B. Airless lungs alters "ee" to sound like "ay" |
| C. Asymmetric chest movements | C. ↓ filling of affected lung |
| D. Arterial blood gases | D. May show signs of hypoxia |
| E. Chest x-ray and/or bronchoscopy | E. Visualizes obstructions |
| F. Sputum, viscosity, amount | F. May cause obstruction |
| **III. Administer:** | |
| A. O₂ as ordered | A. Maintain O₂ of tissues |
| B. Analgesics as ordered | B. For relief of pain, avoid respiratory depressant |

## IV. Perform/Provide:

A. Coughing, deep breathing q 2 hr and PRN
B. Postural drainage QID and PRN
C. Nasotracheal suction as ordered
D. Nebulization as ordered with IPPB
E. Semi-Fowler's position

F. Ambulate as soon as possible

A. Stimulates productive cough, promotes O₂
B. Promotes drainage
C. ↓ secretions
D. ↓ viscosity
E. ↓ dyspnea, lowers diaphragm, increases lung expansion
F. Aids in expulsion of secretions

## V. Teach patient/family:

A. Avoid smoking
B. Basic knowledge about disease process and test
C. Need for influenza immunization if over 60
D. Symptoms to report URI, flu, dyspnea, persistent cough
E. Avoid OTC medications
F. Avoid fatigue

A. ↓ air exchange
B. Familiarity reduces anxiety
C. ↓ potential for complications
D. Atelectasis may recur
E. May depress respirations
F. Exercise increases need for O₂

---

**CONCEPT/NEED:** Inflammation/Infection

**NURSING DIAGNOSIS:** Potential infection related to increased secretions

**GOAL:** Absence of infection as evidenced by: temperature WNL, nonpurulent sputum

## INTERVENTION

## RATIONALE

## I. Monitor, describe, record:

A. Temperature q 4 hr and PRN

A. Sign of infection

## II. Assess for:
A. Sputum, flushed, seizures    A. Bacteria or viral infections

## III. Administer:
A. Antibiotics    A. Prevents or destroys growth of microorganisms

B. Antipyretics    B. ↓ abnormally high temperature

## IV. Perform/Provide:
A. Institute strict medical asepsis    A. Prevents cross-infection

B. Tepid sponge bath    B. ↓ temperature

## V. Teach patient/family:
A. Avoid persons with infections (URI)    A. ↓ cross-infection

B. Name of medications, dosage, time to administer, purpose, and side effects    B. Insures safe administration

C. Need to report elevation in temperature and sputum production    C. Sign of infection

---

**CONCEPT/NEED:** Fluid balance

**NURSING DIAGNOSIS:** Potential fluid volume deficit related to low intake of fluids

**GOAL:** Adequate fluid volume as evidenced by: good skin turgor, maintaining weight, ability to raise secretions

## INTERVENTION

## RATIONALE

### I. Monitor, describe, record:
A. I&O q 8 hr    A. Indicates fluid balance

### II. Assess for:
A. Current fluid status    A. Needed for data base

## IV. Perform/Provide:

A. FF to 3000 ml/day unless contraindicated

A. Prevents dehydration, keeps secretions liquid

## V. Teach patient/family:

A. Drink at least 12 glasses of fluid/day

A. Prevents dehydration

# ■ Bronchitis/Bronchiectasis/Asthma

**DEFINITION:** Bronchitis (chronic) is the diffused or localized inflammation of the bronchial tree characterized by cough and large amounts of sputum. Bronchiectasis is the chronic dilation of the bronchi causing destruction of the elastic and muscular structures and secretion of purulent sputum. Asthma is the spasm or swelling or the bronchi causing dyspnea and wheezing as a result of antigen-antibody hypersensitivity reactions

**CONCEPT/NEED:** Oxygenation

**NURSING DIAGNOSIS:** Impaired gas exchange related to bronchial inflammation

**GOAL:** Adequate gas exchange as evidenced by: respirations 16–20, deep, even, clear sputum, lungs clear to auscultation bilaterally

| INTERVENTION | RATIONALE |
|---|---|
| **I. Monitor, describe, record:** | |
| A. Breath sounds q 2–4 hr. Respiration rate and quality | A. Diminished or absent over affected area, wheezing |
| B. Cough, amount and appearance of sputum | B. If sputum separates in 3 layers, indicates bronchiectasis |
| **II. Assess for:** | |
| A. Shortness of breath, cyanosis, restlessness | A. ↓ O₂ supply |
| B. Respiratory status to include history and physical assessment | B. Needed for data base |
| C. Auscultation of chest rales, hyperresonance, inspiratory and expiratory wheeze and rhonchi | C. S&S of asthma, air retention |
| D. Arterial blood gases | D. May reflect respiratory acidosis/hypoxia |
| E. Chest x-ray and/or bronchoscopy | E. Hyperinflation of alveoli |

F. Sputum

F. Eosinophils, Charcot-Leyden crystals in asthma

G. CBC

G. Leukocytosis, ↓ Hct and Hgb in asthma, polycythemia

H. Pulmonary function tests, spirometry

H. ↓ vital capacity, forced expiratory volume, ↑ residual volume

I. Dizziness, hemoptysis, gastric distention

I. Complications of IPPB, bronchodilators

J. Flaring nostrils, prolonged expiration with wheezing, cyanosis, air hunger

J. ↑ respiratory distress

K. Mental confusion, lethargy, semi-coma

K. ↑ $CO_2$ level

L. Chronic or recurrent cough

L. Productive in bronchitis, dry in asthma

M. Shortness of breath, audible expiratory wheeze

M. Result of bronchospasm in asthma

N. Barrel chest, elevated shoulders, flattened molar bones, narrow nose, distended neck veins

N. Continuous trapping of air in the lungs with increased residual capacity

O. Hemoptysis: fetid breath (See Respiratory Assessment, p. 105)

O. Symptom of bronchiectasis

## III. Administer:

A. $O_2$ as ordered

A. Maintain $O_2$ of tissues

B. Antitussives as ordered

B. For relief of nonproductive cough of bronchitis

C. Bronchodilators/expectorants/ liquefying agents

C. Improve ventilation

## IV. Perform/Provide:

A. Diaphragmatic breathing with emphasis of prolonged expiration

A. Stimulates productive cough, ↓ $CO_2$

B. Postural drainage QID and PRN

B. Promotes drainage

C. High humidity environment

C. Liquefies secretions

D. Nebulization as ordered with IPPB

D. Assists in bringing up secretions

E. High Fowler's position

E. Promotes ventilation

## V. Teach patient/family:

| | |
|---|---|
| A. Avoid smoking | A. ↓ gas exchange |
| B. Basic knowledge about disease process and test | B. Familiarity reduces anxiety |
| C. Nasal rather than mouth breathing | C. Nasal breathing warms and filters air |
| D. Assume upright position when dyspneic | D. ↑ gas exchange |
| E. Use humidifier, no flowering houseplants | E. Increases humidity. Flowers cause allergies |
| F. Use of nebulizer, exhale fully, take deep breaths through the mouth while Y tube is closed hold breath for 3–4 sec, inhale slowly | F. ↑ full gas exchange |
| G. Name of medications, dosage and time to administer, purpose, and side effects | G. Insures safety |
| H. Carry ID card for asthmatic with doctor's name and number, diagnosis, medications, dosage, and allergies | H. Prevents complications, for use in emergency |

---

**CONCEPT/NEED:** Inflammation/Infection

**NURSING DIAGNOSIS:** Potential infection related to pooling of secretions

**GOAL:** Absence of infection as evidenced by: temperature WNL, clear nonpurulent sputum

| **INTERVENTION** | **RATIONALE** |
|---|---|
| **I. Monitor, describe, record:** | |
| A. Temperature q 4 hr and PRN | A. Sign of infection |
| **II. Assess for:** | |
| A. Sputum | A. Mucopurulent in bronchitis |
| B. Allergy test | B. Identifies antigens |
| C. Usual temperature | C. Needed for data base |

### III. Administer:
A. Antibiotics as ordered

B. Antipyretics as ordered

C. Steroids as ordered

A. Prevents or destroys growth of microorganisms

B. ↓ abnormally high temperature, promotes comfort

C. ↓ inflammation

### IV. Perform/Provide:
A. Reduce known allergens
B. Strict medical asepsis

A. Respiratory irritants
B. Prevents cross-infection

### V. Teach patient/family:
A. Avoid persons with infections (URI)

B. Name of medications, dosage, time to administer, purpose, and side effects

C. Need to report elevation in temperature

A. ↓ cross-infection

B. Insures safe administration

C. Sign of infection

---

**CONCEPT/NEED:** Anxiety

**NURSING DIAGNOSIS:** Anxiety related to difficult breathing

**GOAL:** Anxiety will be reduced as evidenced by: verbalization, ability to take slow, deep breaths, ability to sleep during night, pulse WNL

### INTERVENTION

### RATIONALE

### II. Assess for:
A. Verbal and nonverbal clues of anxiety

B. Personal resources to cope with stress

C. Responses to information and treatments

D. Fear of suffocation
(See Psychosocial Assessment for further guidelines, p. 31)

A. Patient may be unable to openly communicate. Open communication reduces stress

B. Provides emotional support

C. Treatments and information may increase or decrease anxiety

D. From decreased $O_2$

## IV. Perform/Provide:

| | |
|---|---|
| A. Accepting environment to state feelings | A. Provides emotional support |
| B. Environment that avoids anxiety-producing situations | B. ↓ anxiety |
| C. Referral for counseling for extremely anxious individual | C. May need professional psychiatric intervention |
| D. Encouragement to perform self-care as able | D. Lessens sense of helplessness and emotional trauma |
| E. Ask patient to close eyes and visualize himself/herself breathing calmly (pursed lips) | E. Relaxation reduces anxiety. Helps rid $CO_2$ |

## V. Teach patient/family

| | |
|---|---|
| A. Avoid anxiety-producing situations | A. ↑ shallow breathing |
| B. Importance of communication with significant other | B. Provides for a release of anxiety |

---

**CONCEPT/NEED:** Fluid balance

**NURSING DIAGNOSIS:** Fluid volume deficit related to decreased intake

**GOAL:** Adequate fluid intake as evidenced by: good skin turgor, maintaining WT, ability to raise secretions

## INTERVENTION / RATIONALE

### I. Monitor, describe, record:

| | |
|---|---|
| A. I&O q 8 hr | A. Indicates fluid balance |

### II. Assess for:

| | |
|---|---|
| A. Current fluid status | A. Needed for data base |
| B. WT QD same time, same clothing, same scale | B. Ensures accurate WT |

### IV. Perform/Provide:

| | |
|---|---|
| A. FF to 3000 ml/day unless contraindicated | A. Thins secretions |
| B. Avoid dairy products | B. ↑ viscosity of secretions |

C. Schedule postural drainage at least 1 hr before meals

C. Promotes appetite by more efficient breathing

## V. Teach patient/family:
A. Drink at least 12 glasses of fluid/day unless contraindicated

A. Prevents dehydration

B. Balance rest and activity

B. Prevents overtiring

# ■ Chronic Obstructive Pulmonary Disease

**DEFINITION:** A group of respiratory disorders in which there is a chronic narrowing of the airways caused by obstruction and affecting the air flow into or out of the lungs. Includes bronchitis, bronchiectasis, asthma, and emphysema

**CONCEPT/NEED:** Oxygenation

**NURSING DIAGNOSIS:** Impaired gas exchange related to obstruction

**GOAL:** Adequate gas exchange as evidenced by: lungs clear to auscultation bilaterally, secretions clear in color

| INTERVENTION | RATIONALE |
|---|---|
| **I. Monitor, describe, record:** | |
| A. Breath sounds q 2–4 hr. Respiration rate and quality | A. Indicates rales/wheezing |
| B. BP, apical pulse q 2 hr | B. Needed for cardiac status |
| **II. Assess for:** | |
| A. Shortness of breath, cyanosis, restlessness | A. ↓ $O_2$ supply |
| B. Respiratory status to include history and physical assessment | B. Needed for data base |
| C. Auscultation of chest for audible expiratory wheezing | C. May indicate bronchospasm |
| D. Arterial blood gases | D. Chronic respiratory acidosis detection |
| E. Sputum | E. Eosinophils, Charcot-Leyden crystals in asthma |
| F. RBC, Hgb, Hct | F. Polycythemia from hypoxia (chronic) |
| G. Dizziness, hemoptysis, gastric distention | G. Complications of IPPB, bronchodilators |

H. Flaring nostrils, prolonged expiration with wheezing, cyanosis, air hunger
I. Mental confusion, lethargy, semi-coma
J. Chronic or recurrent cough
K. Shortness of breath, audible expiratory wheeze
L. Barrel chest, elevated shoulders, flattened molar bones, narrow nose, distended neck veins

(See Respiratory Assessment, p. 105)

H. Increased respiratory distress

I. $CO_2$ narcosis

J. Dry in asthma
K. Results of bronchoplasm

L. Continuous trapping of air in the lungs with increased residual capacity

## III. Administer:
A. $O_2$ as ordered on low flow
B. Aerosols

C. Bronchodilators

A. Maintains $O_2$ of tissues
B. Dilates the lumina of air passages in the lungs
C. Improves ventilation

## IV. Perform/Provide:
A. Diaphragmatic breathing with emphasis on prolonged expiration
B. Postural drainage QID and PRN
C. High humidity environment
D. Nebulization as ordered with IPPB
E. Semi-Fowler's position
F. Deep breathing and coughing q 2 hr

A. Stimulates productive cough

B. Promotes drainage

C. ↓ viscosity of secretions
D. ↓ viscosity of secretions

E. Promotes ventilation
F. Raises secretions

## V. Teach patient/family:
A. Avoid smoking
B. Basic knowledge about disease process, tests, and when to seek help
C. Nasal rather than mouth breathing

A. ↓ air exchange
B. Familiarity reduces anxiety

C. Nasal breathing warms, filters air, and prevents bronchospasm

| | |
|---|---|
| D. Assume upright position when dyspneic | D. ↑ air exchange |
| E. Use humidifier, nonflowering houseplants | E. ↑ humidity |
| F. Use of nebulizer, exhale fully, take deep breaths through the mouth while Y tube is closed hold breath for 3–4 sec, inhale slowly | F. ↑ full air exchange |
| G. Name of medications, dosage and time to administer, purpose, and side effects | G. Insures safety |
| H. Carry ID card with doctor's name, number, diagnosis, medications, dosage, and allergies | H. Prevents complications, for use in emergency |

---

**CONCEPT/NEED:** Inflammation/Infection

**NURSING DIAGNOSIS:** Potential infection related to retained secretions

**GOAL:** Absence of infection as evidenced by: temperature WNL, secretions—clear

## INTERVENTION

### RATIONALE

I. **Monitor, describe, record:**
   A. Temperature q 4 hr and PRN     A. Sign of infection

II. **Assess for:**
   A. Sputum     A. Mucopurulent in bronchitis
   B. Respiratory quality     B. ↑ dyspnea in inflammation
   C. Usual temperature     C. Baseline data

III. **Administer:**
   A. Antibiotics as ordered     A. Prevents or destroys growth of microorganisms
   B. Antipyretics as ordered     B. ↓ abnormally high temperature
   C. Steroids as ordered     C. ↓ inflammation

**IV. Perform/Provide:**

A. Prevent smoking in room | A. Respiratory irritants

**V. Teach patient/family:**

A. Avoid persons with infections (URI) | A. ↓ cross-infection

B. Name of medications, dosage, time to administer, purpose, and side effects | B. Insures safe administration

C. Need to report elevation in temperature | C. Sign of infection

---

**CONCEPT/NEED:** Anxiety

**NURSING DIAGNOSIS:** Anxiety related to dyspnea

**GOAL** Anxiety will be reduced as evidenced by: verbalization, ability to breathe deeply, pulse WNL, ability to sleep at night

## INTERVENTION

## RATIONALE

**II. Assess for:**

A. Verbal and nonverbal clues of anxiety | A. Patient may be unable to openly communicate. Open communication reduces stress

B. Personal resources to cope with stress | B. Provides emotional support

C. Responses to information and treatments | C. Treatments and information may increase or decrease anxiety

D. Fear of suffocation (See Psychosocial Assessment, p. 31) | D. From decreased $O_2$

**IV. Perform/Provide:**

A. Accepting environment to state feelings | A. Provides emotional support

B. Environment that avoids anxiety-producing situations | B. ↓ anxiety

C. Referral for counseling for extremely anxious individual | C. May need professional psychiatric intervention

| | |
|---|---|
| D. Encouragement to perform self-care as able | D. Lessens sense of helplessness and emotional trauma |
| E. Ask patient to close eyes and concentrate on visualizing himself/herself breathing calmly and efficiently | E. Relaxation reduces anxiety |

**V. Teach patient/family:**

| | |
|---|---|
| A. Avoid anxiety-producing situations | A. ↑ shallow breathing |
| B. Importance of communication with significant other | B. Provides for a release of anxiety |

---

**CONCEPT/NEED:** Rest/Sleep

**NURSING DIAGNOSIS:** Potential sleep pattern disturbance related to dyspnea

**GOAL:** Adequate sleep pattern as evidenced by: sleeping 6–8 hr/night, verbalization

| **INTERVENTION** | **RATIONALE** |
|---|---|
| **II. Assess for:** | |
| A. Sleep patterns | A. Needed for data base |
| **III. Administer:** | |
| A. Sedatives as ordered | A. Promotes rest |
| **IV. Perform/Provide:** | |
| A. Organize nursing care to disturb as little as possible | A. Promotes rest |
| B. Limit visitors, discourage talking | B. Conserves energy |
| **V. Teach patient/family:** | |
| A. Balance rest and activity | A. Conserves energy |
| B. Rest 2–3× per day | B. Conserves energy |
| C. Avoid OTC medications | C. May interact with drugs |

**CONCEPT/NEED:** Fluid balance

**NURSING DIAGNOSIS:** Fluid volume deficit related to decreased intake

**GOAL:** Adequate fluid volume as evidenced by: absence of edema, good skin turgor, absence of pulmonary rales

### INTERVENTION

I. **Monitor, describe, record:**
   A. I&O q 8 hr

II. **Assess for:**
   A. Current fluid status
   B. WT QD same time, same clothing, same scale

IV. **Perform/Provide:**
   A. Restrict or limit fluids as ordered

V. **Teach patient/family:**
   A. Perform I&O when discharged

### RATIONALE

A. Retention may be sign of right-sided heart failure

A. Needed for data base
B. Ensures accurate WT

A. ↓ copious mucus

A. Insures safety at home

# ■ Fractured Ribs

**DEFINITION:** An injury in which one or more ribs are broken. May be simple or compound with bone splinters protruding from the chest and may lead to hemothorax, pneumothorax, atelectasis, pneumonia, or flail chest

**CONCEPT/NEED:** Oxygenation

**NURSING DIAGNOSIS:** Ineffective breathing pattern related to pain

**GOAL:** Adequate breathing pattern as evidenced by: normal rate and depth of respirations, productive cough

| INTERVENTION | RATIONALE |
|---|---|
| **I. Monitor, describe, record:** | |
| A. Breath sounds q 2–4 hr. Respiration rate and quality | A. May be decreased or absent over area |
| B. BP, apical pulse q 2 hr | B. For cardiac status |
| **II. Assess for:** | |
| A. Chest expansion q 4 hr | A. ↓ $O_2$ supply |
| B. Respiratory status to include history and physical assessment | B. Needed for data base |
| C. X-ray of chest | C. Location of fracture |
| D. Arterial blood gases | D. Acidosis from hypoventilation |
| E. Hemoptysis (See Respiratory Assessment, p. 105) | E. May indicate lung puncture |
| **IV. Perform/Provide:** | |
| A. Semi-Fowler's position | A. Promotes ventilation |
| B. Deep breathing and coughing q 2 hr | B. Prevents pneumonitis |
| **V. Teach patient/family:** | |
| A. Report sudden sharp chest pains dyspnea, vertigo, pallor | A. Pneumothorax is possible |

B. Avoid contact sports, stren-
uous exercise
C. Avoid persons with URI

B. Prevents complications

C. Prevents infection

---

**CONCEPT/NEED:** Pain

**NURSING DIAGNOSIS:** Alteration in comfort: pain related to inflammation

**GOAL:** Increased comfort as evidenced by: verbalization, ease of breathing

## INTERVENTION

## RATIONALE

**II. Assess for:**
   A. Pain and tenderness over site
      of fracture
   B. Effectiveness of pain relief
   C. Chest expansion

A. Needed for data base

B. For pain management
C. Patient will not expand chest
   when in pain

**III. Administer:**
   A. Local anesthetic and analge-
      sics as ordered

A. For relief of pain

**IV. Perform/Provide:**
   A. Turn to unaffected side and
      back
   B. Place necessary items within
      reach

A. Avoids pressure on injury

B. Avoids straining to reach

**V. Teach patient/family:**
   A. Name of medication, dos-
      age, time to administer, pur-
      pose, and side effects

A. Insures safe administration

# ■ Pleurisy/Pleuritis/Pleural Effusion

**DEFINITION:** An inflammation of the visceral and parietal pleurae usually accompanying inflammatory pulmonary diseases or complication of chest trauma, cancer, or pulmonary infarction. May be wet or dry. Pleural effusion (abnormal increase in pleural fluid) accompanies wet pleurisy as well as diseases such as lung cancer or congestive heart failure

**CONCEPT/NEED:** Oxygenation

**NURSING DIAGNOSIS:** Ineffective breathing pattern related to pain

**GOAL:** Adequate breathing pattern as evidenced by: normal rate and depth of respirations

## INTERVENTION

### RATIONALE

**I. Monitor, describe, record:**
   A. Breath sounds q 2–4 hr. Respiration rate and quality
   B. BP, apical pulse q 2 hr

   A. May have reduced respirations, pleural friction rub
   B. Indicates cardiac status

**II. Assess for:**
   A. Pleural friction rub
   B. Respiratory status to include history and physical assessment

   A. Heard on inspiration
   B. Needed for data base

   C. Auscultation of chest

   C. Diminished or absent breath sound over area
   D. Chest x-ray
   E. Sputum
   (See Respiratory Assessment, p. 105)

   D. May reveal mass, fluid
   E. To identify organism

**IV. Perform/Provide:**
   A. Deep breathing and coughing q 2 hr

   A. Prevents pneumonitis

### V. Teach patient/family:
A. Importance of continuing treatment for primary disease

A. Often treatment is D/C when patient feels better

---

**CONCEPT/NEED:** Pain

**NURSING DIAGNOSIS:** Alteration in comfort: pain related to inflammation

**GOAL:** Increased comfort as evidenced by: verbalization, pulse WNL, no grimacing, ability to sleep at night

### INTERVENTION

### RATIONALE

#### II. Assess for:
A. Pain, tenderness, and characteristics

A. Needed for data base

B. Effectiveness of pain relief

B. Needed to evaluate interventions

#### III. Administer:
A. Analgesics as ordered

A. For relief of pain

#### IV. Perform/Provide:
A. Splint the rib cage during coughing

A. Eases pain

B. Apply heat or cold

B. Applies symptomatic relief

C. Fowler's position

C. Promotes respirations

---

**CONCEPT/NEED:** Rest/Sleep

**NURSING DIAGNOSIS:** Sleep pattern disturbance related to pain

**GOAL:** Adequate sleep as evidenced by: sleeping 6–8 hr/night

### INTERVENTION

### RATIONALE

#### II. Assess for:
A. Sleep patterns

A. Needed for data base

**IV. Perform/Provide:**
   A. Organize nursing care to dis-   A. Promotes rest
      turb as little as possible

**V. Teach patient/family:**
   A. Balance rest and activity   A. Prevents fatigue

---

**CONCEPT/NEED:** Fluid balance

**NURSING DIAGNOSIS:** Fluid volume deficit related to decreased intake

**GOAL:** Increased fluid volume as evidenced by: I&O WNL, good skin turgor

## INTERVENTION

## RATIONALE

**I. Monitor, describe, record:**
   A. I&O q 8 hr   A. Indicates fluid status
   B. WT same time, same scale,   B. Insures accurate WT
      same clothing

**II. Assess for:**
   A. Current fluid status   A. Needed for data base

**IV. Perform/Provide:**
   A. Intake of 2–3 L/day   A. Thins sputum

**V. Teach patient/family:**
   A. Continue increased intake of   A. Thins sputum
      fluid after discharge

# ■ Pneumonia

**DEFINITION:** An inflammation of the alveoli resulting in consolidation of the lungs caused by infectious microorganisms. Depending on areas involved, may be termed lobar pneumonia or bronchopneumonia. May also be termed according to causative agent such as viral, bacterial, or chemical pneumonia

**CONCEPT/NEED:** Oxygenation

**NURSING DIAGNOSIS:** Impaired gas exchange related to inflammation

**GOAL:** Adequate gas exchange as evidenced by: normal rate and depth of respirations, effective removal of secretions by productive cough

| INTERVENTION | RATIONALE |
|---|---|
| **I. Monitor, describe, record:** | |
| A. Breath sounds q 2–4 hr. Respiration rate and quality | A. Indicates respiratory status |
| **II. Assess for:** | |
| A. Irritability, restlessness | A. Sign of decreased $O_2$ |
| B. Respiratory status to include history and physical assessment | B. Needed for data base |
| C. Auscultation of chest | C. Diminished or absent breath sound over area |
| D. Chest x-ray | D. Consolidation |
| E. Arterial blood gases | E. May detect hypoxia |
| F. ESR, WBC | F. Increased in pneumonia |
| **III. Administer:** | |
| A. Antitussives as ordered | A. Minimizes cough |
| B. $O_2$ as ordered | B. ↑ oxygenation |
| C. Expectorants | C. Aids in expelling secretions |
| **IV. Perform/Provide:** | |
| A. Humidifier or steam as ordered | A. Humidified air loosens secretions |

B. Position of comfort
C. Postural drainage and percussion QID
D. Maximum rest
E. IPPB or incentive spirometry

F. Deep breathing and coughing q 2 hr
G. Semi-Fowler's position
H. Prevent smoking

B. ↓ demand for $O_2$
C. Promotes drainage

D. ↓ demand for $O_2$
E. Aids in regaining normal lung function
F. Prevents consolidation

G. ↓ dyspnea
H. ↓ $O_2$ in room

## V. Teach patient/family:

A. Basic knowledge about disease process, diagnostic tests, and procedures
B. Use of vaporizer at home
C. Methods of postural drainage
D. Name of medication, dosage, time and purpose, side effects
E. Report dyspnea, persistent cough

A. Knowledge reduces anxiety

B. Raises secretion
C. Promotes drainage

D. Insures safe administration

E. Avoids complications

---

**CONCEPT/NEED:** Pain

**NURSING DIAGNOSIS:** Alteration in comfort: pain related to coughing

**GOAL:** Increased comfort as evidenced by: verbalization, ability to sleep at night, decreased request for pain medication

## INTERVENTION

## RATIONALE

### II. Assess for:
A. Pain characteristics and respirations

B. Effectiveness of pain relief

C. Level of comfort

### III. Administer:
A. Analgesics as ordered

A. Needed for pain relief

B. Needed for effective pain management

C. Needed for pain management

A. For relief of pain

## IV. Perform/Provide:
A. Splint the rib cage during coughing

A. Eases pain

B. Position of comfort

B. Promotes respirations

## V. Teach patient/family
A. Name of medications, dosage, time, purpose, and side effects

A. Helps insure safe administration

---

**CONCEPT/NEED:** Rest/Sleep

**NURSING DIAGNOSIS:** Potential sleep pattern disturbance related to pain

**GOAL:** Adequate sleep as evidenced by: sleeping 6–8 hr/night, verbalization

### INTERVENTION

### RATIONALE

## II. Assess for:
A. Sleep patterns

A. Needed for data base

## III. Administer:
A. Sedatives, avoid respiratory depressants

A. Respiratory depressants will shorten already shallow respiration

## IV. Perform/Provide:
A. Organize nursing care to disturb as little as possible

A. Promotes rest

B. Complete or partial bed bath

B. ↓ energy expenditure

## V. Teach patient/family:
A. Plan 2–3 rest periods/day

A. Conserves energy

---

**CONCEPT/NEED:** Fluid balance

**NURSING DIAGNOSIS:** Fluid volume deficit related to decreased intake

**GOAL:** Adequate fluid volume as evidenced by: good skin turgor, maintaining WT, I&O WNL

| INTERVENTION | RATIONALE |
|---|---|
| **I. Monitor, describe, record:** | |
| A. I&O q 8 hr | A. Indicates fluid balance |
| B. WT same time, same scale, same clothing | B. Insures accurate WT |
| **II. Assess for:** | |
| A. Current fluid status | A. Needed for data base |
| **III. Administer:** | |
| A. Parenteral fluids with electrolytes if ordered | A. May be needed if electrolytes are low |
| **IV. Perform/Provide:** | |
| A. Intake of 2–3 L/day | A. Thins sputum |
| B. Offer small amounts of fluid often, ice chips at bedside | B. Encourages fluids |
| **V. Teach patient/family:** | |
| A. FF to 3 L/day unless contraindicated | A. Maintains hydration |

---

**CONCEPT/NEED:** Infection

**NURSING DIAGNOSIS:** Potential infection related to increased secretions

**GOAL:** Absence of infection as evidenced by: temperature WNL for 24 hr, ability to raise secretions

| INTERVENTION | RATIONALE |
|---|---|
| **I. Monitor, describe, record:** | |
| A. Temperature q 4 hr and PRN | A. Sign of infection |
| **II. Assess for:** | |
| A. Chills | A. Sign of infection |
| B. Respiratory quality | B. ↑ dyspnea in inflammation |
| C. Sputum culture | C. Reveals pneumococcus or other organisms |

### III. Administer:
A. Antibiotics

B. Antipyretics

A. Prevents or destroys growth of microorganisms

B. ↓ abnormally high temperature

### IV. Perform/Provide:
A. Prevent smoking in room
B. Tepid sponge baths for hyperthermia
C. Strict medical asepsis

A. Respiratory irritants
B. ↓ temperature
C. Prevents cross-infection

### V. Teach patient/family:
A. Avoid persons with infections (URI)
B. Name of medications, dosage, time to administer, purpose, and side effects
C. Need to report elevation in temperature

A. ↓ cross-infection
B. Insures safe administration
C. Sign of infection

# ■ Pneumothorax/Hemothorax

**DEFINITION:** Pneumothorax is the escape of air from an injured lung, bulla eruption, or erosion of a lesion into the pleural cavity. Hemothorax is the collection of blood as a result of chest injury caused by lacerations of the lung or torn intercostal vessels into the pleural cavity. Both conditions can be present at the same time (hemopneumothorax)

**CONCEPT/NEED:** Oxygenation

**NURSING DIAGNOSIS:** Ineffective breathing pattern related to compression of lung

**GOAL:** Effective breathing pattern as evidenced by: respirations deep and regular, ABGs WNL, nailbeds pink

| INTERVENTION | RATIONALE |
|---|---|
| **I. Monitor, describe, record:** | |
| A. Breath sounds q 2–4 hr. Respiration rate and quality | A. Indicates respiratory status |
| **II. Assess for:** | |
| A. Dyspnea, cough, tachypnea | A. Respiratory distress |
| B. Respiratory status to include history and physical assessment | B. Needed for data base |
| C. Auscultation of chest | C. Diminished or absent breath sound over area |
| D. Thoracentesis results | D. Presence of serous or serosanguinous fluid |
| E. Tracheal shift. Distended neck veins | E. Indicates tension pneumothorax |
| **III. Administer:** | |
| A. Antitussives as ordered | A. Minimizes cough |
| B. O₂ as ordered | B. ↑ oxygenation |
| **IV. Perform/Provide:** | |
| A. Elevate head of bed 60 degrees | A. Promotes respirations |

B. Maximum rest
C. IPPB

D. Assist out of bed
E. Closed chest drainage

B. ↓ need for $O_2$
C. Aids in regaining normal lung function

D. Prevents falls
E. Reinflates lung

## V. Teach patient/family:

A. Basic knowledge about disease process, diagnostic tests, and procedures

A. Knowledge reduces anxiety

B. Avoid smoking

B. Respiratory irritant

C. Name of medication, dosage, time and purpose, side effects

C. Insures safe administration

D. Report dyspnea, persistent cough, sharp chest pain, redness

D. Avoids complications

E. Avoid persons with URI

E. ↓ chance of infection

F. Avoid OTC medications

F. May depress respirations

G. Avoid stretching or sudden movement

G. Due to chest tube insertion

---

**CONCEPT/NEED:** Transport/Circulation

**NURSING DIAGNOSIS:** Alteration in tissue perfusion related to blood loss

**GOAL:** Increased tissue perfusion as evidenced by: stable VS

## INTERVENTION

## RATIONALE

### I. Monitor, describe, record:

A. Breath sounds q 2–4 hr, respiration rate and quality

A. Diminished or absent over affected area

B. Pulse q 4 hr

B. Tachycardia and weak pulse indicate shock or further bleeding

### II. Assess for:

A. Hemoptysis

A. Observe for after thoracentesis

B. Change in apical pulse (sound and rate)

B. Indicates mediastinal shift

### III. Administer:
  A. Antihypotensives/volume expanders     A. Treats shock

### IV. Perform/Provide:
  A. Immediate pressure at puncture site     A. Prevents shock
  B. Care for chest puncture site after removal of chest tube     B. Prevents wound infection

### V. Teach patient/family:
  A. Report any pain, swelling, or tenderness of puncture wound     A. May indicate infection
  B. Care of chest puncture wound     B. Prevents infection

---

**CONCEPT/NEED:** Anxiety

**NURSING DIAGNOSIS:** Anxiety related to dyspnea

**GOAL:** Relief of anxiety as evidenced by: absence of dyspnea and pain

### INTERVENTION

### RATIONALE

### II. Assess for:
  A. Verbal and nonverbal clues of anxiety     A. Patient may be unable to openly communicate. Open communication reduces stress

  B. Personal resources to cope with stress     B. Provides emotional support
  C. Responses to information and treatments     C. Treatments and information may increase or decrease anxiety
  D. Fear of suffocation (See Psychosocial Assessment for further guidelines, p. 31)     D. From decreased $O_2$

### IV. Perform/Provide:
  A. Accepting environment to state feelings     A. Provides emotional support
  B. Environment that avoids anxiety-producing situations     B. ↓ anxiety

C. Referral for counseling for extremely anxious individual
C. May need professional psychiatric intervention

D. Encourage to perform self-care as able
D. Lessens sense of helplessness and emotional trauma

E. Ask patient to close eyes and concentrate on visualizing himself/herself breathing calmly and efficiently
E. Relaxation reduces anxiety

## V. Teach patient/family:

A. Importance of communication with significant other
A. Provides for a release of anxiety

---

**CONCEPT/NEED:** Pain

**NURSING DIAGNOSIS:** Alteration in comfort: pain related to trauma

**GOAL:** Increased comfort as evidenced by: verbalization, decreased request for pain medication

### INTERVENTION

### RATIONALE

## II. Assess for:

A. Pain characteristics and respirations
A. Needed for pain relief

B. Effectiveness of pain relief
B. Needed for effective pain relief

C. Pain aggravated by activity
C. ↑ need for $O_2$

## III. Administer:

A. Analgesics as ordered
A. For relief of pain

## IV. Perform/Provide:

A. Rest periods
A. Conserves energy

B. Position of comfort
B. Promotes respirations

## V. Teach patient/family:

A. Name of medications, dosage, time, purpose, and side effects
A. Helps insure safe administration

B. Avoid over exertion, heavy lifting
B. Recurrence of condition

C. Increase activity as tolerated
C. Conserves energy

# ■ Pulmonary Edema

**DEFINITION:** Pulmonary congestion resulting from cardiac disease, drug overdose, or other problems resulting in accumulation of fluid in the interstitial spaces or alveoli of the lungs

**CONCEPT/NEED:** Oxygenation

**NURSING DIAGNOSIS:** Ineffective breathing pattern related to fluid accumulation

**GOAL:** Adequate breathing pattern as evidenced by: normal rate and depth of respirations

## INTERVENTION

I. **Monitor, describe, record:**
   A. Breath sounds q 2–4 hr, respiration rate and quality

II. **Assess for:**
   A. Paroxysmal cough, pink or white frothy sputum
   B. Respiratory status to include history and physical assessment
   C. Auscultation of chest
   D. Intense fatigue and dyspnea
   E. Chest x-ray
   F. ABG

III. **Administer:**
   A. Bronchodilators as ordered
   B. $O_2$ in high concentrations as ordered
   C. Morphine as ordered
   D. Diuretics (Lasix)

## RATIONALE

A. Indicates respiratory status

A. Ruptured pulmonary capillaries

B. Needed for data base

C. Bubbling rales, wheezy
D. ↑ energy needed for breathing
E. Pulmonary congestion
F. ↑ $PCO_2$, ↓ $PO_2$, ↓ pH

A. Facilitates respiration
B. Relieves hypoxia

C. Relieves dyspnea
D. ↓ edema

## IV. Perform/Provide:

| | |
|---|---|
| A. Bedrest in high Fowler's position | A. Orthopneic position to favor pooling of blood in dependent body parts |
| B. Deep breathing and coughing q 2 hr | B. Raises secretions |
| C. IPPB | C. Raises secretions |

## V. Teach patient/family:

| | |
|---|---|
| A. Basic knowledge about disease process, diagnostic tests, and procedures | A. Knowledge reduces anxiety |
| B. Avoid smoking | B. Respiratory irritant |
| C. Name of medication, dosage, time and purpose, side effects | C. Insures safe administration |
| D. Report dyspnea, persistent cough | D. Avoids complications |
| E. Avoid persons with URI | E. ↓ chance of infection |
| F. Avoid OTC medications | F. May depress respirations |

---

**CONCEPT/NEED:** Transport/Circulation

**NURSING DIAGNOSIS:** Alteration in cardiac output: decreased, related to fluid loss

**GOAL:** Adequate cardiac output as evidenced by: normal pulse and BP

| INTERVENTION | RATIONALE |
|---|---|
| **I. Monitor, describe, record:** | |
| A. Breath sounds q 2–4 hr. Respiration rate and quality | A. Indicates respiratory function |
| B. Pulse q 4 hr. Apical pulse q 4 hr | B. Tachycardia, galloping apical rhythm |
| C. WT QD with same scale in same clothing, same time | C. Insures accurate WT |
| D. Peripheral pulses q 15 min | D. When rotating tourniquet is used |
| E. I&O q 1–8 hr | E. Indicates fluid status |

## II. Assess for:

A. Skin temperature, cold clammy skin
A. Peripheral vasoconstriction

B. Distended neck veins, peripheral edema, ascites, hepatomegaly
B. Right-sided heart failure

C. ECG and echocardiogram
C. Tachyarrhythmias and ventricular hypertrophy

D. Chest x-ray
D. Enlargement of heart and engorgement of the pulmonary artery

E. Chest pain
E. Myocardial ischemia

F. Distention of jugular veins
F. ↑ venous pressure when sitting at 45 degree angle

G. Fatigue, weakness
G. Poor tissue perfusion

## III. Administer:

A. Diuretics as ordered
A. ↓ blood volume

B. Cardiotonics as ordered
B. ↑ cardiac output

C. Rotating tourniquets as ordered
C. ↓ venous return

D. Phlebotomy as ordered
D. ↓ R ventricular output

E. Sedation as ordered
E. ↓ discomfort of tourniquets

## IV. Perform/Provide:

A. Rotating tourniquets
A. ↓ fluid in vascular compartment

## V. Teach patient/family:

A. Name of medications, dosage, time of administration, purpose, and side effects
A. ↓ complications

B. Purpose of tourniquets if used
B. Knowledge ↓ anxiety

---

**CONCEPT/NEED:** Anxiety

**NURSING DIAGNOSIS:** Anxiety related to dyspnea

**GOAL:** Relief of anxiety as evidenced by: verbalization, pulse WNL, ability to sleep at night

| INTERVENTION | RATIONALE |
|---|---|
| **II. Assess for:** | |
| A. Verbal and nonverbal clues of anxiety | A. Patient may be unable to openly communicate. Open communication reduces stress |
| B. Personal resources to cope with stress | B. Provides emotional support |
| C. Responses to information and treatments | C. Treatments and information may increase or decrease anxiety |
| D. Fear of suffocation (See Psychosocial Assessment for further guidelines, p. 31) | D. From decreased $O_2$ |
| **IV. Perform/Provide:** | |
| A. Accepting environment to state feelings | A. Provides emotional support |
| B. Environment that avoids anxiety-producing situations | B. ↓ anxiety |
| C. Referral for counseling for extremely anxious individual | C. May need psychiatric intervention |
| D. Encouragement to perform self-care as able | D. Lessens sense of helplessness and emotional trauma |
| **V. Teach patient/family:** | |
| A. Importance of communication with significant other | A. Provides for a release of anxiety |

# ■ Pulmonary Tumors

**DEFINITION:** A growth in the lungs that may be benign or malignant, primary or secondary

**CONCEPT/NEED:** Oxygenation

**NURSING DIAGNOSIS:** Impaired gas exchange related to secretions

**GOAL:** Adequate gas exchange as evidenced by: absence of dyspnea, cough

| INTERVENTION | RATIONALE |
|---|---|
| **I. Monitor, describe, record:** | |
| A. Breath sounds q 2–4 hr. Respiration rate and quality | A. Indicates respiratory status |
| **II. Assess for:** | |
| A. Cough | A. Dry progressing to wet |
| B. Respiratory status to include history and physical assessment | B. Needed for data base |
| C. Hoarseness, dysphagic, vocal paralysis | C. Compression of laryngeal nerve |
| D. Lung scan, bronchoscopy, and biopsy | D. Reveals malignant cells |
| E. Chest x-ray, thoracentesis | E. Reveals malignant cells |
| F. Mediastinoscopy and biopsy, exploratory thoractomy | F. Reveals mass and malignant cells |
| **III. Administer:** | |
| A. Bronchodilators as ordered | A. Facilitates respiration |
| B. O₂ therapy | B. Promotes oxygenation |
| C. Antineoplastics if indicated | C. Destroys malignant cells |
| **IV. Perform/Provide:** | |
| A. Elevate head of bed 30 degrees | A. Promotes respirations |

B. Deep breathing and coughing q 2 hr

B. Raises secretions

C. Postural drainage QID, humidification

C. Promotes loosening and removal of secretions

**V. Teach patient/family:**

A. Basic knowledge about disease process, diagnostic tests, and procedures

A. Knowledge reduces anxiety

B. Avoid smoking

B. Respiratory irritant

C. Name of medication, dosage, time and purpose, side effects

C. Insures safe administration

D. Use vaporizer at home

D. $\uparrow$ ease of respirations

---

**CONCEPT/NEED:** Anxiety

**NURSING DIAGNOSIS:** Anxiety related to prognosis

**GOAL:** Relief of anxiety as evidenced by: verbalization, pulse WNL, ability to sleep at night

## INTERVENTION

## RATIONALE

**II. Assess for:**

A. Verbal and nonverbal clues of anxiety

A. Patient may be unable to openly communicate. Open communication reduces stress

B. Personal resources to cope with stress

B. Provides emotional support

C. Responses to information and treatments

C. Treatments and information may increase or decrease anxiety

D. Fear of surgery
(See Psychosocial Assessment for further guidelines, p. 31)

D. May need emotional support

**IV. Perform/Provide:**

A. Accepting environment to state feelings

A. Provides emotional support

B. Environment that avoids anxiety-producing situations

B. ↓ anxiety

C. Referral for counseling for extremely anxious individual

C. May need psychiatric intervention

D. Encouragement to perform self-care as able

D. Lessens sense of helplessness and emotional trauma

E. Ask patient to close eyes and concentrate on visualizing himself/herself breathing calmly and efficiently

E. Relaxation reduces anxiety

## V. Teach patient/family:

A. Importance of communication with significant other

A. Provides for a release of anxiety

---

**CONCEPT/NEED:** Nutrition

**NURSING DIAGNOSIS:** Potential alteration in nutrition: less than body requirements related to fatigue

**GOAL:** Adequate nutrition as evidenced by: eating 6 small feedings/day

**INTERVENTION**

**RATIONALE**

## II. Assess for:

A. Nutritional and activity status to include usual patterns, physical assessment, and interest

A. Needed for data base

B. I&O q 8 hr

B. Indicates hydration

C. WT QD in same clothing, at same time, same scale

C. Insures accurate WT

## III. Administer:

A. Parenteral therapy as ordered

A. Insures hydration

## IV. Perform/Provide:

A. High calorie, high protein diet with supplemental vitamins

A. Promotes tissue regeneration

B. Frequent oral care

**V. Teach patient/family:**
A. Balance rest and activity
B. Eat balanced diet. Sleep in upright position

B. Promotes appetite

A. Avoids fatigue
B. Promotes adequate nutrition. Promotes adequate respirations during sleep

# ■ Tracheostomy

**DEFINITION:** An opening, with tube insertion, from an incision into the trachea at the second, third, or fourth tracheal ring to assist ventilation by allowing air in and out of the lungs

**CONCEPT/NEED:** Oxygenation

**NURSING DIAGNOSIS:** Impaired gas exchange related to secretions

**GOAL:** Effective gas exchange as evidenced by: breath sounds clear on auscultation

| INTERVENTION | RATIONALE |
|---|---|
| **I. Monitor, describe, record:** | |
| A. Respirations q 4 hr and BP q 4 hr | A. Indicates respiratory status |
| B. Auscultate lung fields q 4 hr | B. Indicates abnormal breath sounds |
| **II. Assess for:** | |
| A. Respiratory status including history and physical assessment | A. Needed for data base |
| B. Restlessness, tachypnea, tachycardia, wheezing, stridor, pallor, cyanosis | B. Airway obstruction |
| C. Tracheostomy cuff (present or absent, inflated or deflated), size of tube | C. Insures safety |
| D. Symmetrical expansion of chest | D. Indicates proper chest expansion |
| E. Breath sounds q 1 hr | E. Indicates ventilation |
| F. Sputum, viscosity/amount | F. Prevents obstruction |
| **IV. Perform/Provide:** | |
| A. Suction PRN | A. Maintains patency of airway |
| B. Elevate head of bed 45 degrees | B. Facilitates ventilation |
| C. Humidify air | C. Prevents drying of mucosa |

| | D. Needed if tube is removed |
|---|---|
| D. Tracheostomy obturator taped at bedside, additional tracheostomy set, self-inflating bag with adaptor | |

**V. Teach patient/family:**

| | |
|---|---|
| A. Need to keep stoma covered | A. Aspiration of dust, etc. |
| B. Importance of not smoking | B. Very irritating |
| C. Not to use aerosol sprays | C. Aspiration possible |
| D. Need for humidifier | D. Prevents drying |
| E. Wear ID with doctor's name, number, diagnosis, medications, and allergies, "neck breather" | E. Prevents complications, used in emergency |
| F. Report respiratory distress | F. May indicate complication |
| G. Blowing nose, sucking, gargling, whistling, lifting, swimming must be avoided | G. May dislodge tube, aspirate water |

---

**CONCEPT/NEED:** Infection

**NURSING DIAGNOSIS:** Potential infection related to contamination

**GOAL:** Absence of infection as evidenced by: temperature WNL, aspirate—nonpurulent, stoma—no redness or swelling

### INTERVENTION

### RATIONALE

**II. Assess for:**

| | |
|---|---|
| A. Temperature q 4 hr | A. Infection indicator |
| B. Purulent aspirate | B. Infection indicator |
| C. Stoma for pain, swelling, drainage | C. Infection indicator |

**III. Administer:**

| | |
|---|---|
| A. Antibiotics as ordered | A. Treats infection |

**IV. Perform/Provide:**

| | |
|---|---|
| A. Remove and clean inner cannula q 8 hr PRN | A. Prevents infection |
| B. Clean stoma q 8 hr | B. Prevents infection |

| C. Administer oral hygiene q 2 hr | C. Minimizes infection |
| D. Shower daily directing spray below neck | D. Prevents water in stoma |

**V. Teach patient/family:**

| A. Care of tracheostomy/stoma, suctioning. Use demonstration/return demonstration | A. Knowledge reduces anxiety |
| B. Handwashing prior to cleaning | B. Prevents infection |
| C. Shower daily directing spray below neck | C. Avoids aspiration |
| D. Shave with electric razor | D. Avoids getting lather into stoma |
| E. Need to cover stoma always | E. Avoids aspiration |
| F. Avoid persons with URI | F. Avoids infection |

---

**CONCEPT/NEED:** Anxiety

**NURSING DIAGNOSIS:** Anxiety related to inability to communicate verbally

**GOAL:** Anxiety reduced as evidenced by: communication by writing or using available aids, pulse WNL, ability to sleep at night

### INTERVENTION

### RATIONALE

**II. Assess for:**

| A. Nonverbal clues of anxiety | A. Patient will be unable to verbally communicate |
| B. Personal resources to cope with stress | B. Provides emotional support |
| C. Responses to information and treatments | C. Treatments and information may increase or decrease anxiety |
| D. Fear of suffocation (See Psychosocial Assessment for further guidelines, p. 31) | D. From decreased $O_2$, artificial airway |

**IV. Perform/Provide:**

| A. Accepting environment to state feelings | A. Provides emotional support |

B. Environment that avoids anxiety-producing situations
C. Referral for counseling for extremely anxious individual
D. Encouragement to perform self-care as able
E. Ask patient to close eyes and concentrate on visualizing himself/herself breathing calmly and efficiently

B. ↓ anxiety

C. May need psychiatric intervention

D. Lessens sense of helplessness and emotional trauma

E. Relaxation reduces anxiety

V. **Teach patient/family:**
   A. Avoid anxiety-producing situations
   B. Importance of communication with significant other

A. ↑ ease of breathing

B. Provides for a release of anxiety

---

**CONCEPT/NEED:** Fluid balance

**NURSING DIAGNOSIS:** Fluid volume deficit related to decreased intake

**GOAL:** Adequate fluid volume as evidenced by: ability to raise secretions, intake of 2000 ml/day

**INTERVENTION**

**RATIONALE**

I. **Monitor, describe, record:**
   A. I&O q 8 hr

A. Indicates hydration

II. **Assess for:**
   A. Current fluid status
   B. WT QD same time, same clothing, same scale

A. Needed for data base

B. Ensures accurate WT

IV. **Perform/Provide:**
   A. FF to 2000 ml/day unless contraindicated
   B. Avoid dairy products

A. Thins secretions

B. ↑ viscosity

V. **Teach patient/family:**
   A. Drink 12 glasses of fluid/day unless contraindicated.

A. Thins secretions

# HEMATOPOIETIC SYSTEM STANDARDS

- Hematopoietic System Assessment
- Anemias/Aplastic/Iron or Folic Acid Deficiency/ Pernicious/Hypovolemic/Hemolytic
- Blood/Blood Products Transfusion
- Hemophilia
- Leukemias/Lymphocytic/Monocytic/Myelocytic
- Lymphomas/Hodgkin's and Non-Hodgkin's Diseases
- Multiple Myeloma
- Polycythemia Vera/Secondary/Relative
- Purpura/Vascular/Thrombocytopenia

# ■ Hematopoietic System Assessment

**DEFINITION:** The collection of a data base concerning the hematopoietic system and its functional capabilities to be used in identifying nursing problems related to transport/circulation, oxygenation, nutrition, inflammation

## I. Interview for and record past history:
A. Previous heart conditions, infections, renal disorders, blood transfusions, hemorrhages, radioactive exposure or radiation, chemical agents
B. Family members with cancer, blood dyscrasias, immune disorders
C. Previous surgery of GI tract, renal or other related to blood-forming organs
D. Allergies to foods, drugs, chemicals
E. Smoking and alcohol use per day, how long
F. Occupation and environmental exposure to benzene or other toxic agents
G. Dietary patterns and inclusion of iron and vitamins
H. Bleeding from gums, nose, bruising, or other body parts
I. Fatigue, WT loss, weakness, pain in bones or joints, enlarged nodes
J. Customary medications taken for pain or other medical conditions
K. Past CBC, Hct, Hgb, RBC indices, bleeding and clotting time, electrolytes, Schilling test, Coombs test, iron level, chest x-ray, and flat plate, scans, lymphangiography, bone marrow puncture, lymph node biopsy, and results

## II. Interview for and record present history:
A. Chief complaint
B. Onset, duration, where took place
C. Principal S&S
D. Knowledge of disease, prognosis, procedures, and planned therapy
E. Results of all blood, urine, x-ray, nuclear medicine tests, and procedures done
F. Treatments and medications taken for hematopoietic problem

## III. Inspection/Observation for:
A. VS to include elevated TPR, rate and characteristics, BP, height and WT
B. Fatigue, weakness, anorexia, nausea, headache
C. Ecchymosis or petechiae, bleeding of gums, nose, or other parts

D. Pain in bones or joints, mouth, tongue and describe
E. Skin color, texture, pallor, pruritus, jaundice
F. Activity abilities, appetite, fluid intake

## IV. Palpation for:
A. Size of liver, spleen
B. Lymph node enlargement, tenderness, movement, size and consistency in neck, axilla, and inguinal area
C. Joints for swelling

# ■ Anemias/Aplastic/Iron or Folic Acid Deficiency/Pernicious/ Hypovolemic/Hemolytic

**DEFINITION:** Aplastic anemia is the decreased production of erythrocytes by the bone marrow. Iron or folic acid deficiency anemia is the decreased production of erythrocytes as a result of inadequate intake of iron and folic acid or increased metabolic needs. Pernicious anemia is the decrease in development of erythrocytes as a result of a deficiency of the intrinsic factor needed to absorb $B_{12}$ in the small intestine. $B_{12}$ is needed for erythrocyte formation. Hypovolemic anemia is the loss of large numbers of erythrocytes from extensive or progressive hemorrhaging. The result is a decrease in blood volume and $O_2$-carrying capacity of the blood. Hemolytic anemia is the accelerated destruction of erythrocytes and the failure of the bone marrow to replace them

**CONCEPT/NEED:** Transport/Circulation

**NURSING DIAGNOSIS:** Alteration in tissue perfusion related to reduced RBCs

**GOAL:** Adequate tissue perfusion as evidenced by: normal VS, skin color—pink

| INTERVENTION | RATIONALE |
|---|---|
| I. **Monitor, describe, record:** | |
| A. BP, pulse, respirations q 4 hr and PRN | A. Indicates cardiac status |
| II. **Assess for:** | |
| A. Hematopoietic assessment to include history and inspection | A. Provides baseline date |
| B. Blood transfusion assessment | B. If blood replacement needed |
| C. Palpitations, dyspnea, headache, dizziness, tinnitus, fatigue, tachycardia | C. ↓ Hgb, and $O_2$ delivery |

D. Bleeding from gums, GI
   tract, urinary tract

D. In aplastic anemia

E. Skin color at rest and during
   activities

E. Indicates respiratory status

F. Paresthesia

F. From reduced RBCs

G. Results of serum iron,
   TIBC, transferrin saturation,
   RBC, reticulocyte count,
   bone marrow stain for
   hemosiderin

G. Low in iron deficiency

   Coombs test
   WBC, platelets
   Serum B$_{12}$

   Positive in hemolytic anemia
   Decreased in aplastic anemia
   Decreased in pernicious anemia

## III. Administer:

A. Blood and blood cell replacements as ordered

A. ↑ RBC

B. Hematinic and iron as ordered

B. ↑ Hgb

C. Pyridoxine HCL as ordered

C. For iron deficiency

D. Corticosteroids as ordered

D. Modifies body's immune response in hemolytic/aplastic
   anemia

E. Vitamin B$_{12}$ as ordered

E. Extrinsic factor in pernicious
   anemia

F. Folic acid as ordered

F. Assists in RBC regeneration

G. Platelet transfusion as ordered

G. Arrests bleeding in aplastic anemia

H. Androgens as ordered

H. Stimulates bone marrow function
   in aplastic anemia

## IV. Perform/Provide:

A. Deep breathing

A. ↑ O$_2$ intake

B. Semi-Fowler's position

B. ↑ oxygenation

C. Keep patient warm

C. ↓ need for O$_2$

## V. Teach patient/family:

A. Nap and change position
   slowly

A. ↓ fatigue

B. Basic knowledge about disease process

B. Knowledge reduces anxiety

C. Name of medications, dosage, time, and side effects

C. Insures safety

D. Avoid aspirin-containing products

D. Have anticoagulant properties

E. Inform all physicians of disorder

E. In aplastic anemia

---

**CONCEPT/NEED:** Safety

**NURSING DIAGNOSIS:** Potential for injury related to altered sensation

**GOAL:** Absence of injury as evidenced by: no breaks, burns, or falls

### INTERVENTIONS

### RATIONALE

**II. Assess for:**

A. Brittle spoon-shaped nails, dizziness

A. In pernicious anemia

B. Motor and sensory responses, loss of position, sense

B. Disturbs gait, possible falls

C. Lack of coordination, paresthesia, delirium

C. In pernicious anemia

D. Reactions to transfusions

D. Insures safety

**III. Administer:**

A. Antibiotics as ordered

A. Prevent infection

**IV. Perform/Provide:**

A. Avoid applying external heat

A. May cause burn

B. Use side rails

B. Prevents injury

C. Assist with ambulation

C. Prevents falls

D. Gentle massage for all pressure points

D. Prevents skin breakdown

**V. Teach patient/family:**

A. Change position slowly, sit when dizzy

A. Prevents falls

B. Avoid person with URI

B. Prevents infection

C. Good hygiene

C. Prevents cross-infections

D. Report elevated temp, colds, flu

D. Indicates infection

E. Keep nails short and avoid scratching

E. Prevents infections/bleeding

**CONCEPT/NEED:** Nutrition

**NURSING DIAGNOSIS:** Alteration in nutrition: less than body requirements related to inadequate intake

**GOAL:** Adequate nutrition as evidenced by: normal RBC count, acceptance of $B_{12}$ medication regimen

## INTERVENTION

## RATIONALE

**II. Assess for:**

A. GI status to include history and physical assessment, usual nutritional patterns

A. Need for data base

B. Anorexia, diarrhea, constipation, WT loss

B. S&S of pernicious anemia

C. Mouth and tongue, difficult swallowing, swelling

C. S&S of pernicious anemia/iron deficiency

D. Gastrectomy

D. Lack of intrinsic factor

E. Cheilosis or fissures of lips

E. Iron deficiency

F. Gastric analysis, gastroscopy

F. ↓ volume in pernicious anemia

G. Schilling test

G. Less than 3% excretion of $B_{12}$ in pernicious anemia

**III. Administer:**

A. Supplemental vitamins, iron

A. Needed to replace vitamins

**IV. Perform/Provide:**

A. Well-balanced diet high in iron and $B_6$

A. Iron deficiency

B. Food high in vitamin $B_{12}$ and folic acid

B. Needed for pernicious anemia

C. Frequent oral care

C. Prevents infection

D. FF to 3000 ml/day unless contraindicated

D. Prevents dehydration

E. Avoid very hot, cold, or spicy foods if mouth lesions are present

E. Minimizes discomfort

F. Lubricate lips

F. Helps prevent fissures

## V. Teach patient/family:

A. Basic nutrition and to maintain diet

A. For adequate nutrition

B. Expect color change in stools

B. Iron salts alter color to dark green or black

# ■ Blood/Blood Products Transfusion

**DEFINITION:** Administration of whole blood or blood components or expanders to restore blood volume or replace serum, plasma, red blood cells, platelets or albumin

## INTERVENTION

### I. Monitor, describe, record:
   A. VS, temperature q 1–2 hr or PRN
   B. Drip rate according to calculations q 15 min
   C. Site for infiltration causing pain, swelling, hematoma
   D. Patency of tubing and cannula

### II. Assess for:
   A. Allergies of any kind, previous reactions
   B. Patient knowledge of procedure and why being done
   C. Choice of site in arm or hand
   D. Type of cannula and administration set to use (no smaller than #18G)
   E. Leaks in bag
   F. Symptoms of transfusion reaction, i.e., temperature, chills, hematuria, dyspnea, cyanosis, headache, malaise, vomiting, diarrhea, tachycardia, edema, hemoptysis, urticaria, wheezing

### III. Perform/Provide:
   A. Venipuncture using aseptic technique
   B. Double check of correct blood for correct patient according to policy
   C. Calculation of drip rate/min and time schedule for completion
   D. Stay with patient for 15 min after starting blood
   E. Inform patient to call nurse if any symptoms occur
   F. Change blood tubing and filter according to policy
   G. Comfortable position for patient
   H. Safe removal of cannula after transfusion

# ■ Hemophilia

**DEFINITION:** An inherited bleeding disorder affecting the blood-clotting capability resulting from a deficiency of Factors VIII, IX, or XI in the blood plasma. Affects only males, but is transmitted by females

**CONCEPT/NEED:** Transport/Circulation

**NURSING DIAGNOSIS:** Alteration in tissue perfusion related to bleeding

**GOAL:** Adequate tissue perfusion as evidenced by: Hct and Hgb WNL, absence of frank blood

| INTERVENTION | RATIONALE |
|---|---|
| **I. Monitor, describe, record:** | |
|     A. BP, pulse, respirations q 4 hr | A. Change may indicate bleeding |
| **II. Assess for:** | |
|     A. Hematopoietic assessment to include history and inspection | A. Provides baseline data |
|     B. Hemarthrosis, hematuria, epistaxis, and bleeding after injury or minor surgery | B. Indicates bleeding |
|     C. PTT, Lee-White clotting time | C. Decreased clotting |
| **III. Administer:** | |
|     A. Blood and blood cell replacements (See Blood/Blood Products, Transfusion, p. 160) | A. Provides adequate cells and volume |
|     B. Topical hemostatics as ordered | B. Controls bleeding locally |
|     C. Coagulants | C. Controls bleeding systemically |
|     D. Blood factor as ordered | D. Replaces clotting factor |
|     E. Sedation as ordered | E. Quiets patient during treatment |

## IV. Perform/Provide:
| | |
|---|---|
| A. Pressure on wound | A. ↓ loss of blood |
| B. Immobilize and elevate part | B. Movement increases blood loss |
| C. Apply cold compresses to bleeding site | C. Constricts blood vessels |
| D. Maintain joint immobility during bleeding | D. Prevents hemorrhage |
| E. Rotate IM sites | E. Prevents hemorrhage |

## V. Teach patient/family:
| | |
|---|---|
| A. Measures to control bleeding (see above) | A. Prevents hemorrhage |
| B. Basic knowledge about disease process | B. Knowledge reduces anxiety |
| C. Name of medications, dosage, time, and side effects | C. Insures safety |
| D. Avoid aspirin-containing products | D. Has anticoagulant properties |
| E. Inform all physicians of disorder | E. Prevents complications |
| F. Information about hemophiliac groups | F. Provides emotional support |
| G. Encourage noncontact sports | G. Prevents injury |
| H. Control of WT | H. Excess WT causes stress on joints |

---

**CONCEPT/NEED:** Pain

**NURSING DIAGNOSIS:** Alteration in comfort: pain related to injury

**GOAL:** Increased comfort as evidenced by: verbalization, no grimacing, pulse WNL

## INTERVENTION

## RATIONALE

### II. Assess for:
| | |
|---|---|
| A. Pain and its characteristics | A. Needed for pain relief |

### III. Administer:
| | |
|---|---|
| A. Analgesics as ordered | A. Controls pain |
| B. Sedatives as ordered | B. Promotes rest |

**IV. Perform/Provide:**
  A. Avoid excessive manipulation during nursing care
  B. Use bed cradle

  A. Prevents pain/bruising

  B. Keeps WT off affected area

**V. Teach patient/family:**
  A. Prevent injury

  A. Avoids bruises/pain

# ■ Leukemias/Lymphocytic/ Monocytic/Myelocytic

**DEFINITION:** A malignant disease characterized by overproduction of abnormal or immature leukocytes involving the bone marrow, spleen, and lymph nodes. Classified according to type of white blood cell involved (lymphocytes, monocytes, or granulocytes). May be chronic or acute

**CONCEPT/NEED:** Anxiety

**NURSING DIAGNOSIS:** Anxiety related to prognosis of disease

**GOAL:** Reduction in anxiety as evidenced by: verbalization, ability to sleep at night, pulse WNL

| INTERVENTION | RATIONALE |
|---|---|
| **II. Assess for:** | |
| A. Verbal and nonverbal clues of anxiety | A. Patient may be unable to express feelings openly |
| B. Personal resources to cope with illness | B. Provides emotional support |
| C. Personal response to diagnosis | C. Needed for data base |
| D. Depression, hopelessness, anger, denial, altered body image | D. May need time to resolve |
| E. Ability for home care | E. Home care may reduce anxiety |
| F. Spiritual needs (See Spiritual Assessment, p. 35) | F. Needed for data base |
| G. Wishes regarding visitors | G. May wish to be alone |
| **IV. Perform/Provide:** | |
| A. Comfortable quiet environment | A. ↓ anxiety |
| B. Answer all questions truthfully | B. Fosters trust |

C. Information about home care or hospice

C. Needs planning before D/C

D. Contact family's clergy if requested

D. For spiritual comfort

E. Opportunity for expression of fears, questions and grief

E. Provides support

F. Involvement in patient care by family

F. Allows family to feel control, ↓ guilt

G. Provide privacy, listen and share grief when death occurs

G. Will need emotional support

## V. Teach patient/family:

A. Importance of communication with others

A. Provides sharing

B. About remissions from therapies, prevention of infection

B. Gives incentive to continue

C. About any extraordinary measures used to prolong life

C. May need to make decision regarding this

---

**CONCEPT/NEED:** Transport/Circulation

**NURSING DIAGNOSIS:** Alteration in tissue perfusion related to bleeding

**GOAL:** Adequate tissue perfusion as evidenced by: Hct and Hgb WNL, absence of blood from nose, mouth, petechiae

## INTERVENTION

## RATIONALE

### I. Monitor, describe, record:

A. BP, pulse, respirations q 4 hr and PRN

A. Indicates cardiac status

### II. Assess for:

A. Hematopoietic assessment to include history and inspection

A. Provides baseline data

B. Blood transfusion assessment

B. Provides baseline data

C. Hematuria, epistaxis, and gingival bleeding
D. Dyspnea on exertion
E. WBC, RBC, Hct, platelets, PT, PTT
F. Bone marrow studies
G. Serum uric acid
H. Leukocyte alkaline phosphatase (LAP)
I. Chest x-ray

J. Dragging sensation or enlargement of left side of abdomen

C. ↓ clotting, ↑ bleeding

D. ↓ RBCs, ↓ $O_2$ carrying ability
E. Provides for status and response to treatment
F. Abnormal leukopoietic tissue
G. Elevated
H. Differentiates myelocytic/leukomoid
I. Mediastinal node and lung involvement

J. Splenic enlargement

## III. Administer:
A. Blood cell replacements as ordered
B. Antineoplastics as ordered

A. Replaces cells

B. ↓ malignant cell growth

## IV. Perform/Provide:
A. Pressure on wound
B. Use soft/foam toothbrush or waterpik
C. Flotation mattress, bed cradle, and sheepskin

A. ↓ loss of blood
B. ↓ trauma

C. ↓ irritation, pressure

## V. Teach patient/family:
A. Measures to control bleeding
B. Basic knowledge about disease process
C. Name of medications, dosage, time, and side effects

A. Prevents hemorrhage
B. Knowledge reduces anxiety

C. Insures safety

---

**CONCEPT/NEED:** Infection

**NURSING DIAGNOSIS:** Potential infection related to immunosuppressive drugs

**GOAL:** Absence of infection as evidenced by: normal temperature, CBC WNL, temperature WNL

| INTERVENTION | RATIONALE |
|---|---|

**I. Monitor, describe, record:**
   A. Temperature q 4 hr and PRN    A. Symptom of infection

**II. Assess for:**
   A. Fever, chills, night sweats    A. Symptoms of infection
   B. History of frequent infections, reddened areas on skin    B. Needed for baseline data
   C. Enlarged and tender lymph nodes    C. From local tissue invasion
   D. Inflammation at injection sites, changes in VS, cough, and changes in mucous membranes    D. Indicates infection
   E. Blood, stool, urine, and throat cultures    E. Identifies organism
   F. Concentration of circulating granulocytes    F. May be reduced

**III. Administer:**
   A. Antibiotics as ordered    A. Controls infection

**IV. Perform/Provide:**
   A. Laminar air-flow room    A. Control of contamination
   B. Life-island unit    B. Isolates patient from environment
   C. Exclude visitors or staff with infections    C. Prevents infection
   D. Establish protective isolation if needed    D. Prevents infection
   E. Use povidone-iodine for handwashing before entering room    E. Prevents infection
   F. Good oral, skin, and toileting hygiene    F. Control of contamination

**V. Teach patient/family:**
   A. Avoid persons with infections    A. Prevents infection
   B. Good hygiene    B. Prevents infection
   C. Keep nails short and avoid scratching    C. Microorganisms are under nails
   D. Report elevated temperature, colds, flu, or reddened areas on skin    D. Indicates infection

**CONCEPT/NEED:** Pain

**NURSING DIAGNOSIS:** Alteration in comfort: pain related to disease process

**GOAL:** Increased comfort as evidenced by: verbalization, decreased request for pain medication, ability to sleep at night

| INTERVENTION | RATIONALE |
|---|---|
| **II. Assess for:** | |
| A. Arthralgia and bone pain, sternal tenderness | A. Needed for pain relief |
| B. Abdominal discomfort, oral discomfort | B. Needed for pain relief |
| C. Rectal irritation | C. From disease process |
| D. Burning sensation during infusion | D. Local irritation in vein |
| **III. Administer:** | |
| A. Analgesics as ordered | A. ↓ pain |
| B. Aloe vera products | B. ↓ stomatitis |
| **IV. Perform/Provide:** | |
| A. Antiseptic anesthetic mouthwashes | A. Relieves stomatitis |
| B. Position of comfort | B. Relieves pain |
| C. Handle patient gently when turning | C. Prevents pain |
| D. Flotation mattress, bed cradle, and sheepskins | D. Prevents skin breakdown |
| E. Passive ROM | E. Prevents muscle wasting |
| **V. Teach patient/family:** | |
| A. Name of medications, dosage, time, purpose and side effects | A. Safe administration |

---

**CONCEPT/NEED:** Nutrition

**NURSING DIAGNOSIS:** Alteration in nutrition: less than body requirements related to decreased intake

**GOAL:** Adequate nutrition as evidenced by: eating high caloric diet

| INTERVENTION | RATIONALE |
|---|---|
| **II. Assess for:** | |
| A. GI status to include history and physical assessment, usual nutritional patterns | A. Needed for data base |
| B. Anorexia, constipation, WT loss | B. Needed for data base |
| C. Sore mouth and tongue, difficult swallowing | C. Needed for data base |
| D. Preferences in food selection | D. ↑ appetite |
| E. Gastric ulcers | E. Side effects of prednisone therapy |
| **III. Administer:** | |
| A. Supplemental vitamins | A. Needed when anorexia is present |
| **IV. Perform/Provide:** | |
| A. Bland diet high in iron | A. ↓ nausea, provides nutrients |
| B. Small attractive frequent feedings | B. Small meals stimulate appetite |
| C. Frequent oral care | C. ↓ anorexia |
| D. Avoid very hot, cold, or spicy foods if mouth lesions are present | D. May cause nausea, pain |
| E. Lubricate lips | E. Avoids cracking |
| **V. Teach patient/family:** | |
| A. Basic nutrition and to maintain diet | A. Insures nutrition |

# ■ Lymphomas/Hodgkin's and Non-Hodgkin's Diseases

**DEFINITION:** A group of malignant diseases of the lymphoid system. They are classified according to cell differentiation and origin of the malignant cell. Hodgkin's originates in the lymph nodes, non-Hodgkin's in the lymphatic tissues as well as lymph nodes

**CONCEPT/NEED:** Anxiety

**NURSING DIAGNOSIS:** Anxiety related to prognosis

**GOAL:** Reduction in anxiety as evidenced: verbalization, pulse WNL, ability to sleep at night

| INTERVENTION | RATIONALE |
|---|---|
| **II. Assess for:** | |
| A. Verbal and nonverbal clues of anxiety | A. Patient may be unable to express feelings openly |
| B. Personal resources to cope with illness | B. Needed for data base |
| C. Patient's personal response to diagnosis | C. May need emotional support |
| D. Depression, hopelessness, anger, denial, altered body image | D. May need time to accept these feelings, may indicate grieving |
| E. Ability for home care | E. Home care may reduce anxiety |
| F. Spiritual needs (See Spiritual Assessment, p. 35) | F. Needed for data base |
| G. Wishes regarding visitors | G. May wish to be alone |
| **IV. Perform/Provide:** | |
| A. Comfortable quiet environment | A. ↓ anxiety |
| B. Answer all questions truthfully | B. Fosters trust |

C. Information about home care or hospice
C. Needs pre-planning

D. Contact family's clergy if requested
D. For spiritual comfort

E. Opportunity for expression of fears, questions, and grief
E. Provides support

F. Involvement in patient care by family
F. May provide control, ↓ guilt

G. Provide privacy, listen and share grief when death occurs
G. Provides emotional support

## V. Teach patient/family:

A. Importance of communication with others
A. Allows for sharing

B. About remissions from therapies
B. Gives incentive to continue

---

**CONCEPT/NEED:** Nutrition

**NURSING DIAGNOSIS:** Potential alteration in nutrition: less than body requirements related to decreased intake

**GOAL:** Adequate nutrition as evidenced by: maintenance of weight gain, good appetite, absence of vomiting

## INTERVENTION

## RATIONALE

### I. Monitor, describe, record:
A. I&O q 8 hr
A. Indicates fluid balance

B. WT QD
B. Indicates nutritional status

### II. Assess for:
A. Nutritional status to include history and physical assessment
A. Provides baseline data

B. WT loss, fatigue, vomiting/nausea
B. Indicates possible fluid/nutritional imbalance

C. Dehydration or edema of extremities
C. Increased metabolic rate, increased pressure on veins

D. Favorite foods
D. ↑ food intake

## III. Administer:
A. Antiemetics as ordered      A. ↓ vomiting

## IV. Perform/Provide:
A. FF to 3000 ml/day unless contraindicated      A. Maintains fluids

B. Diet high in calories, proteins, minerals      B. Maintains nutrition

## V. Teach patient/family:
A. Maintain fluids      A. Prevents dehydration

B. Basic knowledge about disease process      B. Knowledge reduces anxiety

C. Name of medication, dosage, time, and side effects      C. Insures safety

---

**CONCEPT/NEED:** Infection

**NURSING DIAGNOSIS:** Potential infection related to immunosuppressive medications

**GOAL:** Absence of infection as evidenced by: temperature WNL, WBC WNL

## INTERVENTION      RATIONALE

### I. Monitor, describe, record:
A. Temperature q 4 hr and PRN      A. Symptom of infection

### II. Assess for:
A. Fever, chills, night sweats      A. Symptoms of infection

B. History of frequent infections, reddened areas on skin      B. Needed for data base

C. Enlarged/tender lymph nodes      C. Local tissue invasion

D. Inflammation at injection sites, changes in VS, cough, and changes in mucous membranes      D. May indicate infection

E. Blood, stool, urine and throat cultures      E. Identifies organism

F. Concentration of circulating granulocytes   F. ↑ in lymphomas

G. Hepatosplenomegaly   G. Enlarged in these disorders

H. Pruritis   H. Bile is deposited on skin

## III. Administer:
A. Antibiotics as ordered   A. Controls infection

## IV. Perform/Provide:
A. Laminar air-flow room   A. Control of contamination

B. Life-island unit   B. Isolates patient from environment

C. Exclude visitors or staff with infections   C. Prevents infection

D. Establish protective isolation if needed   D. Prevents infection

E. Use povidone-iodine before entering room   E. Prevents infection

F. Good oral, skin, and toileting hygiene   F. Control of contamination

G. Lotion to back and pressure areas   G. Prevents skin breakdown

H. Antipruritic lotions   H. Relieves itching

## V. Teach patient/family:
A. Avoid persons with infections   A. Prevents infection

B. Good hygiene   B. Controls contamination

C. Keep nails short and avoid scratching   C. Microorganisms are under nails

D. Report elevated temperature, colds, flu, or reddened areas on skin   D. Indicates infection

# ■ Multiple Myeloma

**DEFINITION:** A malignant disease characterized by plasma cell invasion of the bone marrow and soft tissues leading to disruption in the production of erythrocytes, leukocytes, and thrombocytes

**CONCEPT/NEED:** Pain

**NURSING DIAGNOSIS:** Alteration of comfort: pain related to calcium loss

**GOAL:** Relief of pain as evidenced by: verbalization, decreased request for pain medication, pulse WNL

| INTERVENTION | RATIONALE |
|---|---|
| **II. Assess for:** | |
| A. Arthralgia and bone pain, sternal tenderness | A. ↑ calcium loss |
| B. Pathological fractures | B. ↑ calcium loss |
| C. Renal calculi | C. Demineralization of bone |
| D. Spinal cord compression | D. Tumor size change |
| E. Limitations on activity caused by pain | E. Needed to reduce pain |
| F. Pain characteristics, location, response to activity, and pain relief measures | F. Needed to reduce pain |
| **III. Administer:** | |
| A. Analgesics as ordered | A. ↓ pain |
| **IV. Perform/Provide:** | |
| A. Antiseptic anesthetic mouthwashes | A. Relieves stomatitis |
| B. Position of comfort | B. Relieves pain |
| C. Handle patient gently when turning | C. Prevents pain |
| D. Flotation mattress, bed cradle, and sheepskins | D. Prevents pressure |

## V. Teach patient/family:

A. Name of medications, dosage, time, purpose, and side effects

A. Safe administration

B. Report increased pain in body part

B. Possible fracture

---

**CONCEPT/NEED:** Nutrition

**NURSING DIAGNOSIS:** Potential alteration in nutrition: less than body requirements related to decreased intake

**GOAL:** Adequate nutrition as evidenced by: eating 6 small meals/day, absence of vomiting

### INTERVENTION

### RATIONALE

## II. Assess for:

A. GI status to include history and physical assessment, usual nutritional patterns

A. Needed for data base

B. Anorexia, vomiting, constipation, WT loss

B. Possible fluid imbalance

C. Sore mouth and tongue, difficult swallowing

C. Painful to take fluids

D. I&O q 8 hr

D. Indicates fluid balance

E. Preferences in food selection

E. ↑ nutritional status

F. Urine—Bence Jones protein

F. Positive in this disorder

G. Serum calcium, serum uric acid

G. ↑ in this disorder

H. Proteinuria, hypercalciuria

H. ↑ in this disorder

## III. Administer:

A. Supplemental vitamins

A. Insures all vitamins

B. Allopurinol as ordered

B. ↓ uric acid

C. Diuretics, phosphates, corticosteroids

C. ↓ hypercalcemia

D. Antiemetics as ordered

D. ↓ anorexia/vomiting

## IV. Perform/Provide:

| | |
|---|---|
| A. Bland diet high in iron | A. Less painful to eat, iron needed to rebuild tissues |
| B. Small attractive frequent feedings | B. ↓ anorexia |
| C. Frequent oral care | C. For comfort |
| D. FF to 3000 ml/day unless contraindicated | D. Insures fluids |
| E. Avoid very hot, cold, or spicy foods if mouth lesions are present | E. May injure tissue, cause pain |

## V. Teach patient/family:

| | |
|---|---|
| A. Basic nutrition and to maintain diet | A. Insures proper nutrition |
| B. Maintain fluid intake | B. Minimizes hypercalcemia |

---

**CONCEPT/NEED:** Infection

**NURSING DIAGNOSIS:** Potential infection related to immunosuppressive drugs

**GOAL:** Absence of infection as evidenced by: temperature WNL, no chills

### INTERVENTION

### RATIONALE

**I. Monitor, describe, record:**

| | |
|---|---|
| A. Temperature q 4 hr and PRN | A. Symptom of infection |

**II. Assess for:**

| | |
|---|---|
| A. Fever, chills, night sweats | A. Symptoms of infection |
| B. History of frequent infections | B. Needed for data base |
| C. Enlarged and tender lymph nodes | C. From local tissue invasion |
| D. Inflammation at injection sites, changes in VS, cough, and changes in mucous membranes | D. Symptoms of infection |
| E. Blood, stool, urine, and throat cultures | E. Identifies organism |

|   | F. Indicates infection |
| --- | --- |
| F. Concentration of circulating granulocytes | |

## III. Administer:
| | |
| --- | --- |
| A. Antibiotics as ordered | A. Controls infection |
| B. Prophylactic gamma globulin | B. Supplements depressed immunological system |

## IV. Perform/Provide:
| | |
| --- | --- |
| A. Exclude visitors or staff with infections (protective isolation) | A. Prevents infection |

## V. Teach patient/family:
| | |
| --- | --- |
| A. Avoid persons with infections | A. Prevents infection |
| B. Good hygiene | B. Prevents infection |
| C. Keep nails short and avoid scratching | C. Microorganisms are under skin |
| D. Report elevated temperature, colds, flu, or reddened areas on skin | D. Indicates infection |

# ■ Polycythemia Vera/ Secondary/Relative

**DEFINITION:** Polycythemia vera is the unrestricted increase of erythrocyte production by the bone marrow resulting in increased viscosity and total volume of blood causing congestion of blood in tissues. Secondary polycythemia is the increase of erythrocyte production in response to hypoxemia from a disease such as chronic obstructive pulmonary disease or prolonged exposure to high altitudes that require an increase in $O_2$ demand by the body. Relative polycythemia is the increase of erythrocyte production relative to body plasma loss resulting from fluid loss and dehydration caused by diarrhea, vomiting, or diuretics

**CONCEPT/NEED:** Transport/Circulation

**NURSING DIAGNOSIS:** Alteration in tissue perfusion related to increased blood viscosity

**GOAL:** Adequate tissue perfusion as evidenced by: RBC WNL, absence of chest pain or shortness of breath

| INTERVENTION | RATIONALE |
|---|---|
| **I. Monitor, describe, record:** | |
| A. BP q 4 hr and PRN. Pulse q 4 hr and PRN | A. Indicates cardiac status |
| **II. Assess for:** | |
| A. Hematopoietic assessment to include history and inspection | A. Provides baseline data |
| B. Ruddy complexion, pruritis, CHF | B. Symptoms of disorder |
| C. Chest pain, tachycardia, shortness of breath | C. Symptoms of disorder |
| D. Enlarged spleen and liver | D. Engorgement of blood |
| E. WBC, RBC, Hct, Hgb, platelet count | E. ↑ in this disorder |

F. Leukocytes, alkaline phosphatase, serum uric acid

F. ↑ in this disorder

G. Hypotension during phlebotomy

G. Blood loss, ↓ BP

H. Thrombotic complications, intermittent claudication, MI, CVA

H. From increased viscosity of blood

I. Hemorrhage in any organ system

I. Engorgement of capillary beds

### III. Administer:

A. Radioactive isotopes as ordered

A. Suppresses hemopoietic activity

B. Myelosuppressive alkylating agents

B. Suppresses hemopoietic activity

C. Phlebotomy—repeated until Hct is below 50%

C. Reduces blood volume

D. Radiation to spleen and bone marrow

D. Reduces production of RBCs/pressure on spleen

### IV. Perform/Provide:

A. Diet limiting intake of iron

A. ↓ RBCs

B. Reposition patient q 2 hr

B. ↓ congestion

### V. Teach patient/family:

A. Avoid meats, eggs, legumes, nuts, grains

A. ↓ RBCs

B. Basic knowledge about disease process

B. ↓ anxiety

C. Name of medication, dosage, time, and side effects

C. Insures safety

D. Radiation will not harm others

D. ↓ anxiety

E. Possibility of regular blood donations rather than phlebotomy

E. ↓ blood volume

---

**CONCEPT/NEED:** Oxygenation

**NURSING DIAGNOSIS:** Impaired gas exchange related to increased viscosity of blood

**GOAL:** Adequate gas exchange as evidenced by: ABGs WNL, respirations WNL, ability to perform activities without shortness of breath

| INTERVENTION | RATIONALE |
|---|---|
| **I. Monitor, describe, record:** | |
| A. Respirations q 4 hr | A. Indicates respiratory status |
| **II. Assess for:** | |
| A. Orthopnea, dyspnea on exertion | A. ↓ $O_2$ |
| B. Arterial blood gases | B. Indicates $O_2$ level |
| C. URI | C. ↓ respirations |
| **IV. Perform/Provide:** | |
| A. Elevate head of bed | A. ↓ dyspnea |
| B. Turn, cough, and deep breathe q 4 hr | B. ↓ dyspnea |
| C. Rest periods | C. ↓ $O_2$ need |
| **V. Teach patient/family:** | |
| A. Deep breathing exercises | A. ↑ lung expansion |

---

**CONCEPT/NEED:** Fluid balance

**NURSING DIAGNOSIS:** Fluid volume deficit related to inadequate fluid intake

**GOAL:** Adequate fluid volume as evidenced by: 3000 ml/day of fluid

| INTERVENTION | RATIONALE |
|---|---|
| **II. Assess for:** | |
| A. Thirst | A. Indicates reduced fluids |
| B. I&O q 8 hr | B. Indicates fluid status |
| **IV. Perform/Provide:** | |
| A. FF to 3000 ml/day unless contraindicated | A. ↑ fluids |
| **V. Teach patient/family:** | |
| A. Maintain fluid intake | A. ↓ blood viscosity |

# ■ Purpura/Vascular/ Thrombocytopenia

**DEFINITION:** The bleeding into skin, tissues, and mucous membranes resulting from vascular damage (vascular) or platelet deficiency (thrombocytopenia). The small hemorrhages are called petechiae, the larger are called ecchymoses

**CONCEPT/NEED:** Transport/Circulation

**NURSING DIAGNOSIS:** Alteration in tissue perfusion related to decreased platelet count

**GOAL:** Adequate tissue perfusion as evidenced by: platelets WNL, absence of petechiae, ecchymosis, epistaxis

| INTERVENTION | RATIONALE |
|---|---|
| **I. Monitor, describe, record:** | |
| A. BP q 4 hr and PRN, pulse q 4 hr and PRN | A. Indicates cardiac status |
| **II. Assess for:** | |
| A. Hematopoietic assessment to include history and inspection | A. Provides baseline data |
| B. Skin hemorrhages, menorrhagia | B. Possible hemorrhage |
| C. GI bleeding, hematuria, epistaxis | C. Indicates bleeding |
| D. Petechiae, ecchymosis | D. Indicates bleeding |
| E. RBC, Hct, Hgb, platelet count | E. ↓ in this disorder |
| **III. Administer:** | |
| A. Prednisone as ordered | A. Suppresses antibody formation |
| B. Myelosuppressive agents | B. Used if prednisone does not work |
| C. Blood and blood products | C. Needed for hemorrhage |
| D. Progesterone-estrogen agents | D. Suppresses menstrual flow |

## IV. Perform/Provide:

A. Care after splenectomy (See Post-Op Care, p. 17)

A. Prevents complications

B. Use smallest bore needles

B. Reduces bleeding tendencies

C. Flotation mattress, sheepskins, foam gel pads, bed cradle

C. Avoids skin trauma

D. Use fingersticks for lab work

D. Bleeding tendencies

## V. Teach patient/family:

A. Avoid exposure to infections

A. Chance of infection

B. Basic knowledge about disease process

B. ↓ anxiety

C. Name of medications, dosage, time, and side effects

C. Insures safety

D. Not to donate blood

D. ↓ blood volume

E. Use sharp objects carefully

E. Avoids trauma

F. Inspect for abrasions, hematomas QD

F. Insures safety

G. Pre-op teaching for splenectomy

G. ↓ anxiety

---

**CONCEPT/NEED:** Pain

**NURSING DIAGNOSIS:** Alteration in comfort: pain related to pressure

**GOAL:** Increased comfort as evidenced by: verbalization, decreased request for pain medications

## INTERVENTION

## RATIONALE

### II. Assess for:

A. Pain

A. Needed for data base

B. Headache

B. Possible cerebral hemorrhage

### III. Administer:

A. Analgesics other than aspirin

A. ↓ pain

## IV. Perform/Provide:
A. Swabs for mouth care      A. Avoids trauma
B. Position of comfort      B. Prevents pain
C. Handle patient gently when turning      C. Prevents pain
D. Back massage      D. ↑ comfort

## V. Teach patient/family:
A. Name of medications, dosage, time, purpose and side effects      A. Safe administration

B. Report increased pain in body part      B. Possible fracture, possible hemorrhage

# ENDOCRINE SYSTEM STANDARDS

- Endocrine System Assessment
- Addison's Disease
- Cushing's Syndrome
- Diabetes Insipidus
- Diabetes Mellitus
- Hyperparathyroidism/Hypoparathyroidism
- Hyperthyroidism/Hypothyroidism
- Thyroidectomy

# ■ Endocrine System Assessment

**DEFINITION:** The collection of a data base concerning the endocrine system and its functional capabilities to be used in identifying nursing problems related to hormonal balance/imbalance

## INTERVENTION

### I. Interview and investigate for and record past history:
   A. Previous cardiovascular, pancreatic, renal conditions, psychological problems, obesity
   B. Family members with diabetes, cancer, thyroid disease, hypertension
   C. Previous surgery on thyroid, adrenal, or other glands or any exposure to radiation
   D. Allergies to foods, drugs, or chemicals
   E. Years as a diabetic, diet and insulin therapy
   F. Ability to follow diabetic regimen
   G. Changes in WT, stamina, libido, mental status, muscle activity, respirations, pulse, elimination pattern, appetite, temperature, urinary output, fluid intake, thirst, skin color, fat distribution
   H. Weakness, fatigue, bone pain, palpitations, shortness of breath, frequent infections, edema, visual disturbances, menstrual disorders
   I. Customary medication taken for pain or other medical conditions (prescribed and OTC)
   J. Past urinalysis, CBC, BMR, $T_3$, $T_4$, TSH, ACTH, iodine uptake, electrolytes, cholesterol, blood glucose, ketones, BUN, ABGs, cortisol and other hormones, 17-ketosteroids, scans

### II. Interview and investigate for and record present history:
   A. Chief complaint
   B. Onset, duration, where took place
   C. Principal S&S
   D. Knowledge of disease, prognosis, procedures, and planned therapy
   E. Results of all blood, urine, radiological tests and procedures and treatments done
   F. Medications taken for existing endocrine problem

### III. Inspection for:
   A. VS to include changes in respiration and pulse rate, depth, dyspnea, increased or decreased temperature, height and WT changes

B. Skin color, turgor, dryness, oiliness, texture, edema, nail texture, hair amount, distribution, texture, odor of breath, fat distribution
C. Polyuria or oliguria, thirst, polydipsia, anorexia, constipation, vomiting, diarrhea
D. Muscle weakness, twitching, spasms, fatigue, numbness, tingling, cramping
E. Nervousness, irritability, drowsiness, confusion, depression, anxiety, headache, syncope
F. Moon face, protruding eyeballs, thickening of tongue, hoarseness, bone pain
G. Activity, sleep and other life style patterns

## IV. Palpation for:
A. Thyroid gland
B. Decrease or absence of reflexes
C. Edema, skin texture, temperature, dryness

# ■ Addison's Disease

**DEFINITION:** An adrenocortical insufficiency resulting from the destruction of or sudden cessation in functioning of the adrenal cortex causing deficiencies of aldosterone and cortisol and androgens.

**CONCEPT/NEED:** Fluid balance

**NURSING DIAGNOSIS** Fluid volume deficit related to increased urinary output

**GOAL:** Adequate fluid volume as evidenced by: intake 3000 ml/day, electrolytes WNL, good skin turgor

## INTERVENTION

I. Monitor, describe, record:
   A. BP q 4 hr and PRN
   B. WT QD with same clothing at same time
   C. I&O q 8 hr

   D. Hourly urines

II. Assess for:
   A. Serum chemistries and electrolytes
   B. Skin turgor

   C. Urine specimen for 17-ketosteroids (17-ks), 17-hydroxycorticoids, and 17-ketogenic steroids
   D. Plasma cortisol
   E. Fall in systolic pressure, weak pulse, and cold clammy skin
   F. Moon face, dependent edema, pulmonary edema, and cerebral edema

## RATIONALE

A. Hypotension due to hyponatremia
B. WT gain may indicate impending renal failure
C. Decreased urine output may indicate impending renal failure
D. Identify drop in urine output

A. ↓ sodium and chloride, ↑ potassium and BUN
B. Poor turgor is a sign of dehydration
C. All values decreased

D. No response to ACTH
E. S&S of Addisonian crisis

F. Excessive fluids, sodium and/or adrenal hormones

| G. Muscle weakness, flaccidity, and cardiac arrhythmias | G. Signs of hypokalemia. Most are hyperkalemic |

### III. Administer:

| A. Normal saline infusions as ordered | A. Corrects hypovolemia |
| B. Glucocorticoids and mineralocorticoids as ordered | B. Replaces deficient or absent adrenocortical hormones |
| C. Vasopressors as ordered | C. For severe hypotension |
| D. Volume expanders | D. For decreased BP |

### IV. Perform/Provide:

| A. High sodium, low potassium diet as ordered | A. Helps control electrolyte balance |
| B. FF intake to 3000 ml/day | B. Prevents dehydration |
| C. Place sign in patient's bathroom during 24-hour urine collection | C. Prevents uninformed family or personnel from disposing of urine |

### V. Teach patient/family:

| A. Basic knowledge about disease process, treatments, and tests | A. ↑ compliance for lifelong therapy |
| B. Maintain fluid intake as ordered | B. Prevents dehydration |
| C. Name of medication, purpose, dosage and time to administer | C. Insures safety |
| D. Carry injectable steroid | D. For crisis |
| E. Wear Medic-Alert ID | E. Specify Addison's disease/taking steroids in case of emergency |

---

**CONCEPT/NEED:** Nutrition

**NURSING DIAGNOSIS:** Alteration in nutrition: less than body requirements related to anorexia

**GOAL:** Adequate nutrition as evidenced by: absence of nausea, vomiting, eating all meals, taking nutritious snacks

| INTERVENTION | RATIONALE |
|---|---|

**II. Assess for:**

A. Nutritional status to include 24-hr diet recall and physical assessment — A. Needed for data base

B. Nausea and vomiting, anorexia and WT loss — B. S&S of Addisonian crisis

C. Abdominal pain, diarrhea, or constipation — C. S&S of Addisonian crisis

D. Basic metabolic rate (BMR) — D. ↓ BMR in this disease

E. Fasting blood sugar — E. Hypoglycemia

F. Patency of nasogastric tube — F. Prevents gastric distention and vomiting

**III. Administer:**

A. Antiemetics as ordered — A. For control of nausea, vomiting

**IV. Perform/Provide:**

A. High carbohydrate, high protein diet — A. Prevents WT loss

B. Frequent small feedings — B. May be better tolerated

C. Between meal snacks — C. ↑ caloric intake

D. Give largest dose of cortisone therapy with food — D. ↓ nausea

**V. Teach patient/family:**

A. Avoid dieting without medical supervision — A. May lead to crisis

---

**CONCEPT/NEED:** Anxiety

**NURSING DIAGNOSIS:** Anxiety related to inability to cope with stress

**GOAL:** Decreased anxiety as evidenced by: patient stating stress reduced, pulse WNL, ability to plan activities to reduce stress

| INTERVENTION | RATIONALE |
|---|---|

**II. Assess for:**

A. Verbal and nonverbal clues of anxiety — A. Patient may be unable to express feelings openly

B. Apathy, irritability and emotional instability
C. Reduced libido and loss of secondary sex characteristics
D. Increased stress from work, family life, or other source
E. Increase anxiety due to need for lifelong medication
(See Psychosocial Assessment, p. 31)

B. Indicates stress
C. Indicates adrenal insufficiency
D. Addisonian crisis may be precipitated by stress
E. Change in body image

## IV. Perform/Provide:
A. Comfortable quiet environment
B. Encourage participation in self-care as allowed by activity restrictions
C. Limit visitors that upset patient
D. Explanations about equipment, treatments, and personnel

A. ↓ anxiety
B. Lessens sense of helplessness and emotional trauma
C. Reassurance reduces anxiety
D. ↓ anxiety

## V. Teach patient/family:
A. Avoid stressful situations
B. Importance of communication with significant other
C. Importance of need to deal with significant other

A. ↓ chance of crisis
B. Provides for a release of tension and anxiety
C. ↓ stress and fear of sexual ability and performance

# ■ Cushing's Syndrome

**DEFINITION:** A condition resulting from overactivity of the adrenal gland or administration of synthetic glucocorticoids causing hypersecretion or high level of glucocorticoids

**CONCEPT/NEED:** Fluid balance

**NURSING DIAGNOSIS:** Fluid volume excess related to decreased urinary output

**GOAL:** Fluid balance as evidenced by: normal serum electrolytes, absence of edema, BP WNL

## INTERVENTION

I. **Monitor, describe, record:**
   A. I&O q 8 hr
   B. BP q 4 hr and PRN

   C. WT QD on same scale with same clothing at same time

II. **Assess for:**
   A. Endocrine assessment to include history and physical assessment
   B. Headaches
   C. Muscular weakness
   D. Nocturia and polydipsia

   E. Pitting edema of ankles
   F. Serum potassium and serum sodium
   G. Serum chloride
   H. Intravenous urography
   I. Adrenal scan
   J. Dexamethasone suppression test

## RATIONALE

A. Indicates fluid status
B. Hypertension due to hypervolemia and hypernatremia
C. Fluid retention due to sodium retention increases WT

A. Needed for data base

B. Due to hypertension
C. Due to hypokalemia
D. Diminished response to antidiuretic hormone (ADH)
E. Hypervolemia, ↑ sodium
F. ↓ potassium, ↑ sodium

G. ↓ chloride
H. Adrenal enlargement
I. Possible small adrenal tumors
J. Detects presence of neoplasms

K. ACTH stimulation test

K. Increase in urinary 17-KS and 17-OHCS levels

L. Metyrapone test

L. 17-OHCS levels will fail to rise in presence of neoplasm

M. CAT scan

M. Reveals adenomas and adrenal hyperplasia

N. Daily urine for C&A

N. Increase results from increased glucocorticoids

## III. Administer:

A. Electrolyte replacements particularly potassium as ordered

A. Replaces electrolytes

B. Adrenocortical inhibitors as ordered

B. Inhibits production

C. Adrenal hormone replacement therapy as ordered following total adrenalectomy

C. Glucocorticoid and mineralocorticoid therapy

## IV. Perform/Provide:

A. Explanation about 24-hr urine specimen and sign in bathroom

A. ↑ patient compliance and informs others that urine is to be saved

B. Post-operative care for patient undergoing adrenalectomy

B. (See Post-Operative Care, p. 17)

C. Lift edematous extremities with palms rather than fingers

C. Avoids tissue trauma

## V. Teach patient/family:

A. Never reduce medication dosage or discontinue use without medical supervision

A. Severe rebound of disease process may occur

B. Report delayed healing, ulcers, edema, headaches, and muscle cramps

B. Indicates adverse reactions from medication

C. Importance of wearing a medical alert bracelet

C. Insures safety in emergency

---

**CONCEPT/NEED:** Infection

**NURSING DIAGNOSIS:** Potential infection related to decreased immune response

**GOAL:** Absence of infection as evidenced by: WBCs WNL, temperature WNL

| INTERVENTION | RATIONALE |
|---|---|
| **I. Monitor, describe, record:** | |
| A. Temperature q 4 hr and PRN | A. Indicates infection |
| **II. Assess for:** | |
| A. History of staphylococcal and tuberculous infections | A. Decreased lymph node size, decreased antibody production due to cortisol |
| B. Impaired wound healing | B. From steroids |
| C. Complications, e.g., congestive heart failure and CVA | C. From Cushing's syndrome |
| D. Urinary 17-hydroxycortico-steroids | D. ↑ levels in this disorder |
| E. Plasma 17-hydroxycortico-steroids | E. Diurnal cycle is decreased or absent |
| F. Plasma cortisol | F. ↑ plasma cortisol in this disorder |
| G. Glucose tolerance test | G. Reveals glycosuria and glycemia |
| **IV. Perform/Provide:** | |
| A. Noninfectious environment | A. ↓ infection |
| B. High protein, low calorie, low sodium, and high potassium diet as ordered | B. High protein to prevent muscle wasting, low calorie to reduce WT, low sodium to prevent fluid retention, and high potassium to prevent hypokalemia |
| C. Post-operative wound care and strict asepsis | C. ↓ susceptibility to infection |
| **V. Teach patient/family:** | |
| A. Maintain diet as ordered | A. Needed to reduce symptoms |
| B. Avoid individuals with infections | B. ↑ susceptibility to infection |

---

**CONCEPT/NEED:** Self-image

**NURSING DIAGNOSIS:** Disturbance in self-concept related to increased weight

**GOAL:** Improved self-image as evidenced by: involvement with others, verbalization, planning day's activities

## INTERVENTION

**II. Assess for:**
- A. Verbal and nonverbal clues of anxiety
- B. Moon face, pendulous abdomen, supraclavicular fat pads, heavy trunk, thin extremities
- C. Purple striae

- D. Easy bruising
- E. Muscle wasting, continued decreased ability
- F. Sleeplessness
- G. Acne, hirsutism, recession of hair, breast atrophy, deepened voice, menstrual changes, decreased libido, and impotence

- H. Kyphosis, backache
- I. Mood swings from depression to mania
- J. Urinary 17-ketosteroids
- K. CBC
  (See Psychosocial Assessment, p. 32)

**IV. Perform/Provide:**
- A. Comfortable quiet environment
- B. Stay with patient during periods of emotional crisis
- C. Provide explanations about equipment, surgery, treatments, and personnel
- D. Opportunity for discussions of changes in self-image due to hirsutism and fat deposits

## RATIONALE

- A. Patient may be unable to express feelings openly
- B. Abnormal fat distribution due to increased cortisol

- C. Loss of elastic fibers due to catabolic action of cortisol
- D. Increased fragility of vessels
- E. Elevated cortisol levels

- F. May lead to psychotic behavior
- G. Elevated level of 17-ketosteroids (weak androgen), continued increase masculinization

- H. Due to osteoporosis
- I. Emotional problems increase with decrease in cortisol levels
- J. Increased in urine
- K. Increase in RBC, increase in WBC, decrease in lymphocytes

- A. ↓ anxiety
- B. Provides emotional support
- C. Reassurance reduces anxiety

- D. Fosters open communication

E. Accept patient's behavior and fears, advise that cushingoid symptoms should subside after 4–6 months of treatment

E. Reassurance reduces anxiety

F. Reassurance that emotional symptoms will subside with therapy

F. ↓ anxiety and depression in both patient and family

## V. Teach patient/family:

A. Document psychotic behavior

A. Medication may need to be altered

B. Importance of communication with significant other regarding self-image and sexuality

B. Open communication reduces tension and anxiety

# ■ Diabetes Insipidus

**DEFINITION:** A disorder in the function of the pituitary gland causing a deficiency of the antidiuretic hormone (ADH) resulting in polydipsia and polyuria

**CONCEPT/NEED:** Fluid balance

**NURSING DIAGNOSIS:** Fluid volume deficit related to increased fluid output

**GOAL:** Adequate fluids as evidenced by: good skin turgor, balanced fluid intake and output

## INTERVENTION

I. **Monitor, describe, record:**
   A. I&O q 8 hr
   B. Specific gravity of urine

   C. WT QID with same clothing and scale, same time

II. **Assess for:**
   A. Minimal perspiration
   B. Skin turgor q 4 hr
   C. Urinary 17-ketosteroids and 17-hydroxycorticosteroids and plasma cortisol

III. **Administer:**
   A. Vasopressin as ordered
   B. Parenteral fluids as ordered

IV. **Perform/Provide:**
   A. Adequate fluids
   B. Easy access to bathroom

## RATIONALE

A. Increased up to 10 L/day
B. Decreased specific gravity 1.001–1.005
C. WT loss

A. Increased urine output
B. ↓ turgor, ↑ dehydration
C. Low levels rise slowly after ACTH administration

A. ↓ water loss
B. If unable to tolerate oral fluids

A. May need up to 20 L/day
B. Frequent urination is common, furniture may impede route to bathroom

C. Basic knowledge about disease process, treatments, and tests

D. Maintain fluid intake as ordered

E. Avoid alcohol, coffee, and tea

C. ↑ compliance for lifelong therapy

D. Prevents dehydration

E. Inhibits ADH

# ■ Diabetes Mellitus

**DEFINITION:** A disorder characterized by the inadequate production of insulin by the pancreas to meet body needs for carbohydrate metabolism and resulting in the long-term complications of vascular changes, retinopathy, and neuropathy

**CONCEPT/NEED:** Nutrition

**NURSING DIAGNOSIS:** Alteration in nutrition: more than body requirements related to increased intake

**GOAL:** Adequate intake as evidenced by: eating only items on diet, urine testing WNL, ability to plan diet

## INTERVENTION

**I. Monitor, describe, record:**
- A. WT QD at same time with same clothing, same scale
- B. Pulse q 4 hr

**II. Assess for:**
- A. Polyuria and nocturnal enuresis in children
- B. Polydipsia
- C. Polyphagia
- D. Fatigue, weakness, and lethargy
- E. Skin turgor
- F. Abdominal pain, nausea, and vomiting
- G. Sweet fruity, acetone odor to breath
- H. Stupor, decreased level of consciousness
- I. Diarrhea
- J. Fasting blood sugar

## RATIONALE

- A. Insures accurate WT

- B. Weak, irregular in hypokalemia

- A. S&S of hyperglycemia

- B. S&S of hyperglycemia
- C. S&S of hyperglycemia
- D. S&S of hyperglycemia

- E. Detection of dehydration
- F. S&S of ketoacidosis

- G. S&S of ketoacidosis

- H. S&S of ketoacidosis

- I. S&S of ketoacidosis
- J. 300 mg/100 ml or higher in ketoacidosis

K. Urinalysis

K. Ketonuria in presence of keto-acidosis

L. Blood serum studies

L. $\downarrow$ pH, ketone bodies, $\uparrow$ K and Cl in ketoacidosis

M. Blood gases

M. $\downarrow$ in $P_{CO_2}$

N. Palpitations, weakness

N. S&S of hypokalemia

### III. Administer:
A. Parenteral fluid therapy as ordered

A. For diabetic ketoacidosis to replace sodium

B. Potassium as ordered

B. Replaces potassium loss

C. Insulin as ordered

C. Needed for CHO metabolism

### IV. Perform/Provide:
A. Diet planned according to patient's weight and activities

A. Positive correlation between obesity and diabetes

B. Snacks with carbohydrates in midafternoon and at bedtime

B. $\downarrow$ insulin reaction

C. Encouragement to begin or maintain exercise program

C. Exercise promotes metabolism of CHO, $\downarrow$ insulin requirements

### V. Teach patient/family:
A. Increased food intake, decreased activity, and exercise may lead to ketoacidosis

A. $\uparrow$ metabolism

B. Maintain balanced diabetic diet, exercise and medication as ordered

B. Increase in exercise decreases need for insulin

C. Drink 6–8 glasses of water daily

C. Maintain fluid balance

D. Insulin administration, foot care, urine testing

D. Insures compliance

---

**CONCEPT/NEED:** Infection

**NURSING DIAGNOSIS:** Potential infection related to break in skin integrity

**GOAL:** Absence of infection as evidenced by: no cuts on feet, proper foot care

| INTERVENTION | RATIONALE |
|---|---|

**I. Monitor, describe, record:**

A. Temperature q 4 hr and PRN — A. May indicate infection

B. BP, pulse q 4 hr and PRN — B. Indicates vascular status

**II. Assess for:**

A. Visual disturbances — A. S&S of hyperglycemia

B. Paresthesia, hypoesthesia — B. May lead to injury of extremities

C. Frequent infections — C. S&S of hyperglycemia

D. Slow healing of cuts or scratches — D. S&S of hyperglycemia

E. Cataract formation — E. Linked to chronic hyperglycemia

F. Retinal detachment and blindness — F. Due to complications from retinal lesions

G. Pyelonephritis — G. ↓ renal blood flow

H. Cardiovascular complications, e.g., angina pectoris, coronary insufficiency, intermittent claudication — H. Arteriosclerotic lesions due to diabetic angiopathy

I. Rubor, no posterior tibial pulse, ulcers upon the foot — I. Predisposing S&S of gangrene

J. Dry, scaly skin, itching, blueness, swelling around varicosities, corns, calluses — J. Indicates poor vascular sufficiency

K. Redness, swelling, pain, abrasions — K. S&S of infections from peripheral vascular insufficiency

L. Knowledge regarding flossing and brushing — L. Use soft bristle brush to decrease cuts

M. Examine mouth for irritated gums, bleeding, and dental caries — M. May increase infection

N. Infections of urinary tract — N. Renal vascular disease

**III. Administer:**

A. Antibiotics as ordered — A. For control of infections

**IV. Perform/Provide:**

A. Night light — A. Prevents accidental bumps

B. Slippers, patient should never walk barefoot — B. Avoids trauma to legs and feet

C. Do not use hot-water bottles or electric heating pads on extremities — C. Avoids trauma, skin sensation to heat may be diminished

D. Bathe feet daily in tepid water

E. Inspect feet daily for calluses, corns, blisters

F. Use powder in the web spaces in toes

G. Wear comfortable well-fitting shoes and clean cotton socks

H. Exercise feet regularly

I. Cut nails straight across

J. Avoid smoking, and use of constricting garments

K. Have eye examinations regularly

L. Follow guidelines to avoid urinary infection
(See Cystitis, p. 279)

D. Hot water should never be used

E. Do not treat on own feet. See a podiatrist

F. Prevents moisture between toes

G. Prevents trauma to foot

H. Promotes circulation

I. Prevents trauma to tissues

J. Promotes circulation

K. Detects visual disturbances

L. From change in pH of urine

# ■ Hyperparathyroidism/ Hypoparathyroidism

**DEFINITION:** Hyperparathyroidism is the oversecretion of parathormone (PTH), which controls the metabolism of calcium phosphate and neuromuscular excitability. Hypoparathyroidism is the undersecretion of PTH by the parathyroid glands, which control the metabolism of calcium, phosphate and neuromuscular excitability

**CONCEPT/NEED:** Fluid balance

**NURSING DIAGNOSIS:** Fluid volume deficit related to increased output

**GOAL:** Adequate fluid volume as evidenced by: normal serum electrolytes, adherence to low or high calcium and phosphate dietary intake, absence of dehydration

| INTERVENTION | RATIONALE |
|---|---|
| **I. Monitor, describe, record:** | |
| A. I&O q 8 hr | A. Indicates urinary status |
| B. Color and any irregularities of urinary output | B. Indicates urinary status |
| C. BP and pulse q 4 hr and PRN | C. Detects cardiac irregularities |
| **II. Assess for:** | |
| A. Usual patterns of eating and elimination | A. Needed for data base |
| B. Urinary frequency | B. In hypoparathyroidism |
| C. Constipation | C. S&S of hyperparathyroidism |
| D. Polydipsia and polyuria | D. S&S of hyperparathyroidism |
| E. Renal colic, hematuria, and gravel urine | E. Increased calcium, continued renal calculi formation |
| F. Anorexia and nausea | F. In hypoparathyroidism |
| G. Serum calcium | G. Decreased in hypoparathyroidism, increased in hyperparathyroidism |
| H. Serum phosphorus | H. Decreased in hypoparathyroidism, increased in hyperparathyroidism |

I. Sulkowitch test

J. Urinary phosphate test

K. Radioimmunoassay of PTH

L. Ellsworth-Howard test

M. Serum chloride
N. Serum PTH
O. Urine calcium
P. Tubular reabsorption of phosphate
Q. Blood urea nitrogen (BUN)

R. Serum creatinine

S. Serum alkaline phosphate

I. Decreased or absent urinary calcium in hypoparathyroidism

J. Decreased urinary phosphate in hypoparathyroidism

K. Decreased or absent level in hypoparathyroidism

L. Phosphaturia after IV administration of PTH in hypothyroidism

M. Increased in hyperparathyroidism
N. Increased in hyperparathyroidism
O. Increased in hyperparathyroidism
P. Decreased in hyperparathyroidism
Q. Normal or decreased in hyperparathyroidism

R. Normal or increased in hyperparathyroidism

S. Increased in hyperparathyroidism

## III. Administer:

A. Electrolytes as ordered for hyperparathyroidism

B. Diuretics as ordered for hyperparathyroidism

C. Aluminum salts as ordered for hyperparathyroidism

D. Estrogen, mithramycin, and experimental calcitonin for hyperparathyroidism

E. Calcium salts as ordered for hyperparathyroidism

F. PTH as ordered for hypoparathyroidism

G. Vitamin D as ordered for hypoparathyroidism

H. Aluminum hydroxide gels as ordered for hypoparathyroidism

I. Chlorthalidone as ordered for hypoparathyroidism

A. Promotes electrolyte balance

B. ↑ calcium excretion

C. ↓ gastrointestinal absorption of calcium

D. ↓ serum calcium concentrations

E. ↑ serum calcium levels

F. Replaces missing parathyroid hormone

G. Facilitates absorption of calcium

H. Bonds phosphorus, ↓ serum phosphate

I. Controls hypoparathyroidism

## IV. Perform/Provide:

| | |
|---|---|
| A. High calcium, low phosphorous diet in hypoparathyroidism | A. Prevents electrolyte imbalance |
| B. Low calcium diet, with increased fluids for hyperparathyroidism | B. ↑ fluids to reduce formation of calculi |
| C. Small frequent feedings in hyperparathyroidism | C. ↓ nausea |

## V. Teach patient/family:

| | |
|---|---|
| A. Basic knowledge about disease process and treatment | A. Insures safety |
| B. Name of medication, time to administer, purpose, and dosage | B. ↑ compliance and helps insure safe administration |
| C. Maintain diet and fluid intake as ordered | C. ↑ compliance |
| D. Dialysis may be needed in hyperparathyroidism | D. ↓ calcium levels |

---

**CONCEPT/NEED:** Safety

**NURSING DIAGNOSIS:** Potential for injury related to falls

**GOAL:** Absence of physical injury as evidenced by: absence of falls, lack of seizures

## INTERVENTION

## RATIONALE

### II. Assess for:

| | |
|---|---|
| A. Tetany, carpopedal spasm, paresthesia, tingling, stiffness | A. Indicates calcium imbalance |
| B. Stridor and wheezing, dyspnea | B. Emergency tracheostomy may be needed |
| C. Muscle and abdominal cramps | C. S&S of hypoparathyroidism |
| D. Visual disturbances, photophobia, blurring, and diplopia | D. S&S of hypoparathyroidism |
| E. Dry, scaly skin, fungal infections | E. S&S of hypoparathyroidism |

F. Headache irritability and insomnia

F. S&S of hypoparathyroidism

G. Skeletal deformities of spine, pelvis, and long bones, shortened stature

G. S&S of hyperparathyroidism, increased PTH, continued bone demineralization and hypercalcemia

H. Thickening of nails

H. S&S of hyperparathyroidism, increased PTH, continued bone demineralization and hypercalcemia

I. Pathological fractures

I. From decreased calcium

J. Complications, e.g., peptic ulcer

J. Increased gastric secretion caused by hypercalcemia

K. X-ray examination

K. Increased density of bones in hypoparathyroidism, decalcification in hyperparathyroidism

## III. Administer:

A. Analgesics as ordered for hyperparathyroidism

A. Relieves bone pain

B. Sedatives and magnesium sulfate as ordered for hypoparathyroidism

B. Controls tetany and/or convulsions

C. Anticonvulsants as ordered

C. Controls seizures

## IV. Perform/Provide:

A. Seizure precautions for patient with hypoparathyroidism

A. Insures safety

B. Quiet comfortable environment

B. ↓ anxiety

C. Bed cradle

C. Relieves pressure on painful extremities from bed linens

D. Warm tea and back rubs

D. Promotes rest, ↓ anxiety

E. Move extremities carefully in the hyperparathyroid patient

E. Prevents pathological fractures

F. Night light

F. Protects from fracture due to falls

## V. Teach patient/family:

A. Behavioral changes result from disorder

A. ↓ anxiety

B. Avoid contact sports, heavy lifting

B. Potential for bone fracture

# ■ Hyperthyroidism/Hypothyroidism

**DEFINITION:** Hyperthyroidism is a condition resulting from an oversecretion of thyroxine or triiodothyronine or both by the thyroid gland which controls metabolism. Hypothyroidism results from an undersecretion of hormones by the thyroid gland

**CONCEPT/NEED:** Fluid balance

**NURSING DIAGNOSIS:** Fluid volume deficit related to increased output

**GOAL:** Fluid balance as evidenced by: good skin turgor, absence of edema

| INTERVENTION | RATIONALE |
|---|---|
| I. Monitor, describe, record: | |
| A. WT QID with same clothing and same scale, same time | A. WT gain in hypothyroidism, WT loss in hyperthyroidism |
| B. I&O q 8 hr | B. WT gain in hypothyroidism |
| II. Assess for: | |
| A. Peripheral edema | A. In both hypo- and hyperthyroidism |
| B. Increase diaphoresis | B. In hyperthyroidism |
| C. Serum $T_4$ | C. Decreased in hypothyroidism, increased in hyperthyroidism |
| D. Radioiodine uptake | D. Decreased uptake with hypothyroidism |
| E. Serum $T_3$ | E. Decreased in hypothyroidism, increased in hyperthyroidism |
| F. Radioimmunoassay of TSH | F. Increased in primary hypothyroidism, decreased secondary pituitary hypothyroidism |
| G. Free thyroxine index | G. Increased in hyperthyroidism |
| H. Serum TSH | H. Decreased in hyperthyroidism |
| IV. Perform/Provide: | |
| A. FF to 3000–4000 ml/day | A. In hyperthyroidism |
| V. Teach patient/family: | |
| A. Maintain fluids as ordered | A. Insures fluid volume |

**CONCEPT/NEED:** Skin integrity

**NURSING DIAGNOSIS:** Impairment of skin integrity related to dryness

**GOAL:** Skin integrity as evidenced by: warm, clear skin, absence of breaks

| INTERVENTION | RATIONALE |
|---|---|
| **I. Monitor, describe, record:** | |
| A. Temperature q 4 hr and PRN | A. Subnormal temperature in hypothyroidism |
| **II. Assess for:** | |
| A. Cold intolerance, pale, cool | A. Hypothyroidism due to decreased circulating thyroid hormone. |
| B. Dry skin, brittle nails, hair loss, coarse hair | B. Hypothyroidism due to decreased circulating thyroid hormone. |
| C. Menorrhagia | C. Hypothyroidism due to decreased circulating thyroid hormone. |
| D. Carotenemic skin with rosy cheeks | D. Hypothyroidism due to decreased circulating thyroid hormone. |
| E. Night blindness | E. Hypothyroidism due to decreased circulating thyroid hormone. |
| F. Paresthesia | F. Hypothyroidism due to decreased circulating thyroid hormone. |
| G. Syncope, stupor, and coma | G. Hypothyroidism due to decreased circulating thyroid hormone. |
| H. Heat intolerance with increased perspiration, flushed skin | H. In hyperthyroidism due to increased circulating thyroid hormone |
| I. Palpitation and arrythmia complications | I. In hyperthyroidism due to increased circulating thyroid hormone. |
| J. Severe tachycardia, high temperature, CNS irritability, and delirium | J. Thyroid storm in hyperthyroidism |
| **III. Administer:** | |
| A. Desiccated thyroid hormone as ordered | A. Replaces absent or decreased circulating thyroid hormone in hypothyroidism. |
| B. Iodine and thiouracil as ordered | B. ↑ synthesis of the thyroid hormone |

C. Eye lubricant as ordered     C. In hyperthyroidism

**IV. Perform/Provide:**
  A. Skin moisturizers
  B. Extra blankets and warm environmental temperature in hypothyroidism
  C. Cool, well-ventilated room in hyperthyroidism
  D. Skin care to pressure points QID and PRN, use sheepskin, foam mattress for unambulatory patient

A. For dry skin
B. Prevents heat loss, promotes comfort

C. Promotes comfort

D. Especially important in hypothyroidism to prevent skin breakdown

**V. Teach patient/family:**
  A. Name of medication, purpose, dosage, time to administer
  B. Not to discontinue medication
  C. Report increased temperature, redness and swelling around tissue injury sites, and/or burning on urination
  D. S&S of hypothyroidism, hyperthyroidism

A. Insures safety

B. Both disease states require lifelong therapy
C. S&S of infection process

D. Either condition may result from excessive medication

---

**CONCEPT/NEED:** Coping

**NURSING DIAGNOSIS:** Ineffective individual coping related to lack of control

**GOAL:** Adequate coping as evidenced by: increase in energy and interest (hypothyroidism), ability to relax (hyperthyroidism)

**INTERVENTION**

**RATIONALE**

**II. Assess for:**
  A. Weakness, fatigue and lethargy, muscle stiffness, and aching

A. In both hypo- and hyperthyroidism

B. Headaches

C. Slow speech, thickened tongue, poor memory, slow cognition

D. Loss of libido with personality change to complacent dull and apathetic

E. Excitability, nervousness, restlessness and irritability in hyperthyroidism, increased libido

F. Anger, frustration over changes in physical appearance

B. In both hypo- and hyperthyroidism

C. In hypothyroidism

D. Due to decreased circulating thyroid hormones in hypothyroidism

E. Increased circulation, thyroid hormone

F. Patient may be unable to cope with changes in physical appearance

## III. Administer:
A. Mild tranquilizers or sedatives as ordered

A. For control of hyperactivity, nervousness in hyperthyroidism

## IV. Perform/Provide:
A. Comfortable quiet environment

A. ↓ anxiety

B. Explanations about equipment, treatments, and stress

B. Reassurance reduces anxiety

C. Limit visitors that cause anxiety and stress

C. Prevents emotional upset

D. Reassurance that exophthalmos will recede with therapy

D. ↓ anxiety

E. Assist with activities and ambulation if muscle tremors and weakness interfere

E. Insures safety

F. Back rubs and warm drinks

F. Promotes relaxation

## V. Teach patient/family:
A. Activity level of patient with hypothyroidism will increase within a few days of therapy

A. Symptoms of disease process are reduced with therapy

B. Hyperactivity, mood swings will subside with therapy for hyperthyroidism

B. ↓ anxiety

# ■ Thyroidectomy

**DEFINITION:** Removal of the total or partial thyroid gland in the treatment of hyperthyroidism or cancer of the thyroid

**CONCEPT/NEED:** Learning

**NURSING DIAGNOSIS:** Knowledge deficit related to pre- and post-operative phase

**GOAL:** Adequate knowledge as evidenced by: demonstrating pre-operative teaching

## INTERVENTION

II. **Assess for:**
   A. Endocrine system assessment to include history and physical assessment
   B. (See Hyperthyroidism/Hypothyroidism for S&S of Hyperthyroidism, p. 208)
   C. Knowledge regarding surgical procedure and disease process
   D. Prior surgeries

   E. Severe tachycardia, high temperature, CNS irritability, and delirium

III. **Administer:**
   A. Iodine or thiouracil therapy as ordered

   B. Thyroid hormone as ordered

IV. **Perform/Provide:**
   A. (See Pre-Operative and Post-Operative Care, p. 13, p. 17)

## RATIONALE

A. Needed for data base

B. Removal of the thyroid gland is a treatment for hyperthyroidism

C. ↓ anxiety

D. Previous experience with post-operative care

E. Signs of thyroid storm. May result from decreased thyroid hormone

A. Used pre-operatively to decrease synthesis of thyroid hormone (iodine increases firmness of thyroid, decreases vascularity)

B. Restores normal levels of thyroid hormone post-operatively

A. For more information

# GASTROINTESTINAL SYSTEM STANDARDS

- Gastrointestinal System Assessment
- Cholecystectomy
- Cholecystitis/Cholelithiasis
- Cirrhosis of Liver
- Colostomy/Ileostomy
- Decompression Gastrointestinal Tubes
- Diverticulosis/Diverticulitis
- Gastric/Duodenal Ulcer
- Gastritis
- Hemorrhoids/Hemorrhoidectomy/Rectal Fissure and Fistula
- Hepatitis
- Hernia/Herniorrhaphy
- Intestinal Obstruction
- Pancreatitis
- Total Parenteral Nutrition/Hyperalimentation
- Ulcerative Colitis/Regional Enteritis

# ■ Gastrointestinal System Assessment

**DEFINITION:** The collection of a data base concerning the gastrointestinal system and its functional capabilities to be used in identifying nursing problems related to nutrition and elimination

## INTERVENTION

I. **Interview and investigate for and record past history:**
   A. Previous gastrointestinal conditions such as colitis, ulcers, enteritis, gallbladder problems, hepatitis, diabetes, hemorrhoids, hernia
   B. Previous surgeries such as gallbladder, gastric, bowel, hepatic, hernia, hemorrhoids
   C. Any vomiting or stools with blood, constipation, diarrhea, changes in characteristics of stool, eructation, heartburn, anorexia, WT changes, nausea, vomiting, bulimia, indigestion, pain in abdomen, dysphagia
   D. Family members with ulcers, diabetes, bowel disorders, hemorrhoids
   E. Allergies to food or medication
   F. Pattern of bowel elimination, when, frequency, characteristics
   G. Presence of ostomy, when done and response, pattern of care
   H. Use of laxatives or enemas (prescribed and OTC)
   I. Pattern of food intake, appetite, likes and dislikes, mealtimes, amount, snacks, ability to feed self. Basic 4 and number of calories, 24-hr recall of usual intake for a day
   J. Cultural, religious, and therapeutic restrictions
   K. Ability to chew foods
   L. Use of weight loss programs and products
   M. Factors affecting dietary and elimination pattern such as age, emotions, inactivity, pain, disease
   N. Customary medications taken for indigestion, nausea, vomiting, and response (prescribed and OTC)
   O. Past blood, urine, radiological tests done and results

II. **Interview and investigate for and record present history:**
   A. Chief complaint
   B. Onset and length of illness, signs and symptoms
   C. Knowledge of disease, procedures, and planned therapy
   D. Medications taken for any gastrointestinal problems

E. Treatments such as nasogastric tube, enemas, special diet

F. Results of CBC, electrolytes, bilirubin, amylase, BUN, stool for occult blood, lipase, glucose, sugar tolerance, endoscopy and biopsy, GI series, GB series, sigmoidoscopy, gastric analysis, flat plate x-ray, scans, and others

## III. Inspection for:

A. Height and WT, frame size, overweight or underweight

B. Body contour, bony prominences evident

C. Skin jaundice, texture, rash, edema of extremities, striae on abdomen or legs, erythema, scars

D. Contour of abdomen, flat, concave, rounded, protruding

E. Symmetry of abdomen, peristalsis, pulsations of abdominal aorta

F. Contour of umbilicus, protrusion

G. Mouth tenderness, stomatitis, teeth, and dentures

H. Anal area for hemorrhoids, bleeding, inflammation, excoriation

I. Nasogastric tube drainage, ostomy drainage

J. Changes in stool, tarry, bloody, gray, chalky, mucus, shreds, foul odor, watery

## IV. Auscultation for:

A. Presence, frequency (5–34/min) and character of bowel sounds (clicks, gurgles, loud, rushing, high pitched) in RLQ

B. Bruits of renal, iliac artery or abdominal aorta

C. Absence of bowel sounds (listen for 3–5 min)

## V. Percussion for:

A. Distention of abdomen, flat will be dull, flatus will be tympanic, fluid will be wave-like and shifting dullness

B. Distention of bladder in suprapubic area for dullness

C. Borders of liver in midclavicular line for dullness

D. Stomach at left lower anterior rib cage for tympany

## VI. Palpation for:

A. Tenderness, masses, herniation, inguinal nodes

B. Tightness, distention, warmth

C. Liver, spleen, kidneys not palpable

D. Skin turgor, temperature

E. Rectal mucosa and muscle tone

# ■ Cholecystectomy

**DEFINITION:** A surgical procedure in which the gallbladder is removed

**CONCEPT/NEED:** Anxiety

**NURSING DIAGNOSIS:** Anxiety related to surgery

**GOAL:** Reduction of anxiety as evidenced by: verbalization, pulse WNL, ability to sleep at night

| INTERVENTION | RATIONALE |
|---|---|
| **II. Assess for:** | |
| A. Prior experience with surgical procedures | A. Experience reduces anxiety |
| B. Verbal and nonverbal clues to anxiety | B. Patient may be unable to express feelings openly |
| C. Anxiety level | C. Learning cannot take place with level of anxiety |
| D. Personal resources to cope with stress, e.g., significant other (See Psychosocial Assessment, p. 31) | D. Provides emotional support |
| **IV. Perform/Provide:** | |
| A. Comfortable quiet environment | A. ↓ anxiety |
| B. Stay with patient during periods of increased anxiety or fear related to upcoming surgery | B. Provides emotional support |
| C. Provide explanations about equipment, personnel, exams, and surgical procedure | C. ↓ fear of unknown, ↓ anxiety |
| D. Instruction in deep breathing, coughing pre-operatively | D. Prevents hypostatic pneumonia (a post-operative complication) |

E. Instruction in splinting of incision during deep breathing, coughing exercises pre-operatively

E. Promotes comfort, ↓ pain

F. Side rails up post-operatively

F. Prevents accidental injury from falls

G. Call light within easy reach post-operatively
(See Post-Operative Care, p. 17)

G. Avoids straining or accidental injury

## V. Teach patient/family:

A. Basic knowledge about disease process
(See Pre-Operative guidelines, p. 13)

A. ↓ anxiety

---

**CONCEPT/NEED:** Pain

**NURSING DIAGNOSIS:** Alteration in comfort: pain related to trauma

**GOAL:** Increased comfort as evidenced by: verbalization, reduced request for pain medication, absence of grimacing

## INTERVENTION

## RATIONALE

### II. Assess for:

A. Characteristics of pain
(See Post-Operative Care, p. 17)

A. Needed for data base

B. Response of pain to pain relief measures

B. Medication may need to be adjusted

### III. Administer:

A. Antispasmodics as ordered

A. Relieves spasm

B. Analgesic as ordered

B. Relieves pain

### IV. Perform/Provide:

A. Pain medication before ambulation, deep breathing or coughing exercises

A. ↓ discomfort of procedures post-operatively

B. Scultetus binder before ambulation if ordered post-operatively

B. ↓ discomfort during ambulation

C. Fasten drainage system to clothing or place in pocket

C. ↓ tension on incision and sutures

D. Diet low in fat and roughage pre-operatively

D. ↓ spasms

E. Pillow to splint incision post-operatively

E. ↓ pain on coughing, deep breathing

V. **Teach patient/family:**
   A. Splint incision when turning, coughing, or deep breathing

A. ↓ pain and tension on incisional site

---

**CONCEPT/NEED:** Transport/Circulation

**NURSING DIAGNOSIS:** Alteration in tissue perfusion related to blood loss

**GOAL:** Adequate tissue perfusion as evidenced by: VS WNL, drainage bile-colored, absence of frank blood

## INTERVENTION

## RATIONALE

I. **Monitor, describe, record:**
   A. BP, pulse and respiration q 4 hr and PRN

   A. Changes in VS may indicate complication such as hemorrhage

   B. I&O q 8 hr

   B. Decreased output may indicate hemorrhage

   C. Drainage from T tube is present

   C. Drainage should be dark brown 500–1000 ml/24 hours initially then decrease

II. **Assess for:**
   A. Nausea and vomiting

   A. Sign of obstruction

   B. Jaundice

   B. Possible obstruction of common bile duct

   C. Clay-colored stools
      (See Cholecystitis/Cholelithiasis, p. 221)
      (See Post-Operative Care, p. 17)

   C. Possible obstruction of common bile duct

### III. Administer:
A. IV fluids and electrolytes as ordered

B. Vitamins K and C, blood transfusion as ordered

C. Protein hydrolysate as ordered

A. Replaces volume lost during surgery

B. Elevates a low prothrombin time

C. Aids in wound healing and prevents liver damage

### IV. Perform/Provide:
A. Low Fowler's position

B. Change outer dressing frequently

A. Facilitates lung expansion and drainage of bile

B. Protects skin around incision/observe for bleeding

### V. Teach patient/family:
A. Name of medication, dosage, time to administer, and purpose

A. Insures safe administration

# ■ Cholecystitis/Cholelithiasis

**DEFINITION:** An inflammation or infection of the gallbladder with or without calculi resulting in obstruction, edema, and a decrease in bile expulsion from the gallbladder

**CONCEPT/NEED:** Infection

**NURSING DIAGNOSIS:** Potential infection related to obstruction

**GOAL:** Absence of infection as evidenced by: temperature WNL, WBC WNL

| INTERVENTION | RATIONALE |
|---|---|
| **I. Monitor, describe, record:** | |
| A. Temperature q 4 hr and PRN | A. Major sign of infection process |
| **II. Assess for:** | |
| A. Gastrointestinal assessment to include history and physical assessment | A. Provides baseline data |
| B. Fever/chills | B. Indicates infection |
| C. Cholecystography | C. Reveals presence of stones |
| D. WBC count | D. ↑ WBC count |
| E. Alkaline phosphatase | E. ↑ alkaline phosphatase |
| F. Serum amylase | F. ↑ serum amylase |
| G. Serum lipase | G. ↑ serum lipase |
| H. SGOT | H. ↑ SGOT |
| I. Serum bilirubin and urine bilirubin | I. ↑ cholelithiasis |
| J. Cholangiography | J. Radiopaque dye is injected so all components of the biliary tree can be observed |
| K. Complications, e.g., peritonitis, cholangitis | K. Ruptured gallbladder, peritonitis, bacterially infected, cholangitis |
| **III. Administer:** | |
| A. Antibiotics as ordered | A. Controls infection |
| B. Antispasmodics as ordered | B. Relieves spasm |

## IV. Perform/Provide:

A. (See Cholecystectomy guideline for information regarding surgical management, p. 217)

A. Excision of gallbladder frequently is used for management of cholecystitis/cholelithiasis

B. Low Fowler's position

B. ↓ pressure RUQ

## V. Teach patient/family:

A. Report reoccurrence of pain and other symptoms

A. Chronic infection and inflammation may cause ruptured gallbladder predisposition to attack after initial attack

B. Name of medication, purpose, dosage, time to administer, and side effects

B. ↑ compliance and helps insure safe administration

C. Basic knowledge about the disease process

C. Insures safety

---

**CONCEPT/NEED:** Nutrition

**NURSING DIAGNOSIS:** Alteration in nutrition: less than body requirements related to food intolerance

**GOAL:** Adequate nutrition as evidenced by: eating all meals, absence of nausea and vomiting

## INTERVENTION

## RATIONALE

### II. Assess for:

A. Nausea and vomiting

A. ↓ appetite

B. Indigestion, belching, feeling of fullness, intolerance of fatty foods

B. Intolerance to food resulting from reduced bile secretion

C. Jaundice

C. Stone in common bile duct causes jaundice

D. WT loss

D. Intolerance of fatty foods, nausea, and vomiting

### III. Administer:

A. Antiemetics as ordered

A. Relieves nausea

B. IV fluids and electrolytes as ordered

B. Replaces electrolyte imbalance

C. Vitamins K and C, blood transfusion as ordered

D. Protein hydrolysate as ordered

C. Elevates a low prothrombin

D. Aids wound healing and prevents liver damage pre-operatively

## IV. Perform/Provide:

A. Low fat diet, low roughage diet

B. Nasogastric tube

C. FF to 2500/ml daily unless contraindicated

A. ↓ spasms

B. Decompresses stomach and reduces vomiting pre-operatively

C. Prevents dehydration

## V. Teach patient/family:

A. Maintain low fat diet as ordered

A. Necessary to keep symptoms under control

# ■ Cirrhosis of Liver

**DEFINITION:** A disease characterized by scarring of the liver as a result of alcoholic intake, hepatitis, drug toxicity, infection, or chronic biliary obstruction

**CONCEPT/NEED:** Fluid balance

**NURSING DIAGNOSIS:** Fluid volume excess related to decreased urinary output

**GOAL:** Decreased fluid volume as evidenced by: abdominal girth WNL, decreased weight

## INTERVENTION

## RATIONALE

I. **Monitor, describe, record:**
   A. WT QID with same clothing and same scale, same time
   B. I&O q 8 hr
   C. Abdominal girth measurement q 4 hr

   A. Sudden WT gain may indicate increased fluid retention
   B. Indicates fluid retention
   C. Assesses ascites

II. **Assess for:**
   A. Gastrointestinal assessment to include history and physical assessment
   B. Usual nutritional patterns, 24-hour diet recall
   C. History of chronic alcoholism

   D. Diet high in CHO, low in proteins
   E. Hepatic enlargement

   F. Ascites, pleural effusion, and peripheral edema

   A. Provides baseline data

   B. Needed for data base

   C. Laennec's (portal) cirrhosis, 80% of patients have history of alcohol abuse
   D. Also predisposes patient to Laennec's cirrhosis
   E. Liver initially enlarged because of infiltration
   F. Increased portal venous pressure, congestion, and fluid escaping into abdominal cavity. Decreased ability of liver to synthesize proteins. Decreased colloidal osmotic pressure

G. Esophageal varices

G. Increased pressure and dilation of the esophageal veins

H. Abdominal pain and feeling of fullness

H. Increased pressure due to ascites

I. Anorexia, nausea, vomiting and weight loss, glossitis, fetid breath

I. Due to ascites, anorexia is increased

J. Serum enzymes, e.g., SGOT, SGPT, isocritic dehydrogenase (ICD)

J. SGOT increased, SGPT increased, ICD normal or slightly increased

K. Alkaline phosphatase

K. Increased alkaline phosphatase

L. Direct serum bilirubin, total serum bilirubin, urine bilirubin

L. All increased above normal

M. Serum albumin, globulin

M. Serum albumin decreased, globulin increased

N. BUN

N. Decreased to less than 10 mg/100 ml with gastrointestinal bleeding greater than 20 mg/100 ml

O. Serum uric acid

O. Increased serum uric acid

P. Serum cholesterol

P. Normal or decreased

Q. Prothrombin time

Q. Increased prothrombin time

R. WBC

R. Decreased in hypersplenism, increased with infection

S. RBC

S. Decreased in hypersplenism or hemorrhage

T. Blood ammonia

T. Increased in hepatic failure

U. Bromsulphalein test (BSP)

U. Less than 5% dye retention in 1 hour

V. Serum creatinine

V. Increased serum creatinine

W. Serum electrolytes

W. Sodium below 135 mg/100 ml, potassium above 5.5 mg/100 ml

X. Liver biopsy

X. Fatty changes with or without fibrosis

Y. Barium swallow and esophagoscopy

Y. Reveal and/or confirm presence of esophageal varices

Z. Liver scan

Z. Enlarged liver initially, later atrophy in advanced disease

## III. Administer:

A. Sengstaken-Blackmore tube as ordered

A. Compresses bleeding esophageal varices

B. Blood and plasma as ordered

C. Salt-poor albumin as ordered

D. Diuretics as ordered

E. Supplemental vitamins and minerals as ordered

F. Electrolytes as ordered

B. Maintains central venous and arterial BP

C. Helps maintain colloidal pressure, decreases edema

D. Reduces edema

E. A, B complex, D, and K due to inability to store them

F. Potassium deficiency

## IV. Perform/Provide:

A. Low sodium, increased CHO, diet with adequate protein and calories as ordered

B. Restricted fluid intake 500 ml/day if ordered

C. Ice chips

D. Ration allowed fluid over waking hours

E. Limit gelatin, onions, and strong cheese

A. Low sodium due to fluid retention

B. Due to fluid retention

C. Minimizes thirst

D. Minimizes thirst

E. High ammonia foods

## V. Teach patient/family:

A. Basic knowledge about disease process

B. Name of medication, dosage, time to administer, purpose, and side effects

C. Keep record of I&O and daily weight

D. Limit fluids

E. Report lethargy, increased abdominal girth, dyspnea

A. Helps increase compliance

B. Insures safe administration

C. Indicates fluid retention

D. Avoids fluid retention

E. S&S of complications

---

**CONCEPT/NEED:** Independence
Rest/Sleep

**NURSING DIAGNOSIS:** Alteration in health maintenance related to impaired mobility. Sleep pattern disturbance related to pain

**GOAL:** Health maintenance increased as evidenced by: participation in daily activities, ability to plan diet and activity. Adequate sleep as evidenced by: sleeping 6–8 hr/night, absence of fatigue

| INTERVENTION | RATIONALE |
|---|---|
| **II. Assess for:** | |
| A. Muscle wasting | A. Decreased anabolics |
| B. Usual patterns of self-care, activity to include hygiene | B. Needed for data base |
| C. Mental status | C. Depression over condition or life style |
| D. Usual patterns of rest and sleep | D. Needed for data base |
| **III. Administer:** | |
| A. Sodium pentobarbital as ordered | A. Relieves agitation |
| **IV. Perform/Provide:** | |
| A. Comfortable quiet environment | A. Promotes rest |
| B. Bedrest with bathroom privileges | B. Promotes rest |
| C. Increase activity and encourage self-care as condition improves | C. Lessens sense of helplessness |
| D. Plan nursing care to give maximum rest periods | D. Promotes rest |
| **V. Teach patient/family:** | |
| A. Importance of rest periods during day | A. Limits fatigue |

---

**CONCEPT/NEED:** Skin integrity

**NURSING DIAGNOSIS:** Impairment of skin integrity related to excretions on skin

**GOAL:** Skin integrity as evidenced by: absence of pressure sores, lack of pruritis

| INTERVENTION | RATIONALE |
|---|---|

**II. Assess for:**
- A. Jaundice/pruritis
- B. Condition of pressure points

A. Bile salts cause itching
B. Prevents skin breakdown

**III. Administer:**
- A. Antibiotics as ordered
- B. Antipruritics as ordered

A. Controls or prevents infections
B. Controls pruritus

**IV. Perform/Provide:**
- A. Lotion for skin
- B. Frequent oral hygiene

- C. Reposition q 2 hr

- D. Bathe without soap
- E. Keep fingernails short

A. Prevents drying and cracking
B. Relieves discomfort due to halitosis, glossitis
C. Relieves pressure points, prevents skin breakdown and infection
D. Prevents drying and cracking
E. Prevents patient from scratching skin

**V. Teach patient/family:**
- A. Avoid persons with URI or other infections
- B. Report any swelling, redness, and pain at site of injury
- C. Report any increase in body temperature

A. Lowered resistance to infection

B. S&S of inflammatory infection process

C. Indicates infection

# ■ Colostomy/Ileostomy

**DEFINITION:** A portion of the colon or ileum that has been brought to the surface of the abdomen for the purpose of diverting the flow of fecal material from an inflamed area, a traumatized area, an obstructed area, or a diseased area of the bowel

**CONCEPT/NEED:** Self-esteem

**NURSING DIAGNOSIS:** Disturbance in self concept related to disfigurement

**GOAL:** Increased self concept as evidenced by: participation in care of ostomy, making plans for home care

| INTERVENTION | RATIONALE |
|---|---|
| **II. Assess for:** | |
| A. Verbal and nonverbal clues to anxiety | A. Patient may be unable to express feelings openly |
| B. Personal resources to cope with stress, e.g., significant other | B. Provides emotional support |
| C. Shock, anger, depression, and grief | C. Grieving is a normal process for ostomy patient |
| D. Fear of loss of sexuality, appeal or rejection by family and friends | D. Due to change in body appearance and self-image |
| E. Level of knowledge concerning disease process, temporary or permanent status of ostomy device, and surgical procedure (See Psychosocial Assessment, p. 31) | E. Patient may hold misconceptions regarding disease or treatment |
| **III. Administer:** | |
| A. Sedatives and tranquilizers as ordered | A. ↓ anxiety and promotes rest |

## IV. Perform/Provide:

| | |
|---|---|
| A. Comfortable quiet environment | A. ↓ anxiety |
| B. Stay with patient during periods of emotional crisis | B. Provides emotional support |
| C. Explanations about equipment, treatments, and personnel | C. Reassurance reduces anxiety |
| D. Opportunity for expression of concerns, fears, and questions | D. Fosters open communication |
| E. Encourage participation in self-care as allowed by activity restrictions, encourage acceptance of stoma | E. Lessens sense of helplessness and emotional trauma |

## V. Teach patient/family:

| | |
|---|---|
| A. Importance of communication with a significant other | A. Provides for a release of tension and anxiety |
| B. Importance of need to deal with fears regarding sexual activity | B. ↓ fear of unknown |

---

**CONCEPT/NEED:** Elimination

**NURSING DIAGNOSIS:** Alteration in bowel elimination: incontinence related to loss of sphincter control

**GOAL:** Adequate elimination as evidenced by: lack of constipation/diarrhea, ability to control stools through diet and irrigation

## INTERVENTION    RATIONALE

### II. Assess for:

| | |
|---|---|
| A. (See Pre-operative Care, p. 13) | A. Colostomy may be ordered for treatment of colitis |
| B. Whether colostomy/ileostomy is temporary or permanent | B. Needed for data base |
| C. Site of stoma(s) (ascending, transverse, or descending) | C. There may be a double stoma |

D. Size and color of stoma

E. Pain, distention of abdomen

F. Physical ability of patient to use commode and to irrigate stoma
(See Post-Operative Care, p. 17)

G. Type of ostomy, size and contour of abdomen to choose correct style of pouch

H. Nutritional status to include foods known to irritate the GI system

D. Determines changes

E. Possible obstruction

F. Encourages self-care

G. Prevents leakage of fecal material

H. Individuals vary in foods that cause diarrhea, gas, and constipation

## IV. Perform/Provide:

A. Diet free of foods known to produce gas, diarrhea, or constipation

B. Irrigation of stoma as ordered
(See Post-Operative Care, p. 17)

A. Will vary from individual to individual

B. Colostomy irrigation is not indicated for all patients

## V. Teach patient/family:

A. Seeds, kernels, peanuts will pass undigested into stoma

B. Ileostomy patients may experience a food blockage. A knee-chest position may dislodge obstruction, if not call physician

A. Presence may alarm patient

B. Ingestion of high-fiber foods or improperly chewed food

---

**CONCEPT/NEED:** Skin integrity

**NURSING DIAGNOSIS:** Impairment of skin integrity related to excretions on skin

**GOAL:** Skin integrity as evidenced by: stoma clear of any irritation

| INTERVENTION | RATIONALE |
|---|---|

**II. Assess for:**

A. Type of stoma

A. Ileostomy drainage contains residual digestive enzymes that increase skin breakdown

B. Irritation from frequent pouch changes

B. Symptom of breakdown

C. Redness, pain, swelling around stoma site

C. S&S of infection

D. Effectiveness of pouch system

D. Leakage from poor fitting pouch increases skin breakdown

E. Bright erythema with papular lesions

E. S&S of peristomal yeast infection

**III. Administer:**

A. Skin barrier product as ordered

A. Protects skin exposed by pouch opening

B. Skin sealant as ordered

B. For use under all tapes applied to skin

**IV. Perform/Provide:**

A. Cleansing of skin around stoma

A. Limits peristomal skin irritation

B. Immediate change of leaking stoma pouch

B. Stool against skin increases irritation

C. Heat lamp as ordered

C. Dries irritated area of skin

**V. Teach patient/family:**

A. Cleanse around stoma BID, PRN

A. Limits peristomal skin irritation

B. Change leaking stoma pouch completely and as soon as possible

B. Prevents irritation and skin breakdown

C. Report any redness, swelling or change in skin around stoma

C. Infection or skin breakdown due to improper cleaning or pouch fit

# ■ Decompression Gastrointestinal Tubes

**DEFINITION:** Catheters or tubes that are inserted through the nose or mouth into the stomach and/or intestine for the purpose of removing fluid and air from the tract following surgery, in cases of obstruction and for diagnosing gastrointestinal conditions. Short tubes are the Levin and Salem sump; long tubes are the Miller–Abbott, Harris, and Cantor

## INTERVENTION

### I. Monitor, describe, record:
A. Amount, character, consistency of gastric drainage
B. Serum electrolytes
C. I&O q 8 hr
D. Rectal temperatures

### II. Assess for:
A. Symptoms of fluid deficit to include dry skin and mucosa, skin turgor, lethargy
B. Condition of skin around nares, lips, mouth, and sore throat
C. Abdominal distention
D. Patency of tubing and appropriate taping to the nose and face
E. Tube placement for drainage
F. Proper functioning of suctioning apparatus/pressure
G. Vomiting if any

### III. Administer:
A. Antacids as ordered

### IV. Perform/Provide:
A. NPO as ordered with ice chips if ordered
B. Irrigation of tube with normal saline as ordered and include in I&O
C. Allowance for movement and turning without dislodging tube
D. Semi-Fowler's position for comfort
E. Oral hygiene q 4 hr or PRN
F. Lubricant to nares
G. Proper pressure on suction apparatus
H. IV fluids/electrolytes as ordered
I. Safe removal of tube per order

## V. Teach patient/family:

A. Why tube is used
B. Why nothing must be taken by mouth
C. Turning, deep breathing, movement in bed
D. How to keep tube in place
E. Report any pain, abdominal discomfort

# ■ Diverticulosis/Diverticulitis

**DEFINITION:** A condition in which there are pouches in the mucosa of the gastrointestinal tract, most commonly in the bowel, caused by increased pressure on the lining of the tract or local weakening of the wall. These pouches can become obstructed and inflamed resulting in diverticulitis

**CONCEPT/NEED:** Pain

**NURSING DIAGNOSIS:** Alteration in comfort: pain related to inflammation

**GOAL:** Increased comfort as evidenced by: verbalization, decreased request for pain medication, absence of grimacing

| **INTERVENTION** | **RATIONALE** |
|---|---|
| II. **Assess for:** | |
| A. Characteristics of pain; cramp-like pain in abdomen in LLQ | A. Obstructed and inflamed diverticula increase pain |
| B. Palpation of bowel | B. Reveals a tender colonic mass, usually in descending sigmoid colon |
| III. **Administer:** | |
| A. Anticholinergics and mild sedatives as ordered | A. Relieves spasms |
| IV. **Perform/Provide:** | |
| A. Semi-Fowler's position | A. Promotes comfort |
| B. Unhurried nursing care and emotional support | B. ↓ anxiety, ↑ comfort |
| V. **Teach patient/family:** | |
| A. Report recurrence of pain | A. Insures safety |

**CONCEPT/NEED:** Elimination

**NURSING DIAGNOSIS:** Alteration in bowel elimination related to diet

**GOAL:** Adequate elimination as evidenced by: lack of constipation/diarrhea

| INTERVENTION | RATIONALE |
|---|---|
| **II. Assess for:** | |
| A. Change in bowel habits, constipation, diarrhea, flatulence | A. Needed for data base |
| B. Rectal bleeding or mucus in stool | B. Due to hemorrhage and scarring of bowel |
| C. Nutritional history to include 24-hr diet recall | C. Low fiber, increased carbohydrate diet, constipation |
| D. Usual patterns of elimination | D. History of constipation may be a causative factor in disease |
| E. Complications, e.g., abdominal distention, absence of bowel sounds on auscultation | E. S&S of intestinal obstruction |
| F. Stools for color, consistency, and frequency | F. Possible occult blood, diarrhea |
| G. Barium enema | G. Presence of diverticula and narrowing of bowel lumen |
| H. Sigmoidoscopy | H. Presence of diverticula and thickening of colon wall |
| **III. Administer:** | |
| A. Lubricant and bulk-forming cathartics as ordered | A. Facilitates elimination, ↓ bulk, softens feces |
| B. Antimicrobials as ordered | B. ↓ bowel bacterial flora |
| C. Cleansing enemas as ordered | C. Supports elimination |
| **IV. Perform/Provide:** | |
| A. Bland, high fiber diet | A. Promotes elimination |
| B. Diet free of corn, nuts, seeded vegetables, or fruits | B. Difficult to digest, become trapped in pouches |
| **V. Teach patient/family:** | |
| A. Basic knowledge about disease process | A. ↑ compliance to dietary regimen |
| B. High fiber, high caloric, high protein diet | B. Promotes health of bowel |

C. Avoid constipation

D. Avoid cold food, large meals, alcohol, acid-producing substances

E. Add prunes, wheat germ, bran, raisins, apples, bananas to diet whenever possible

F. Name of medication, dosage, time of administration, purpose, and side effects

C. Straining at stool may increase diverticula

D. Promotes elimination of acid-producing substances

E. Natural laxatives and bulk-forming foods

F. Insures safe administration

# ■ Gastric/Duodenal Ulcer

**DEFINITION:** An ulceration with loss of tissue in the mucosa of the stomach or duodenum believed to be caused by an increase in secretion of acid and gastric juices, stress, or hereditary factors

**CONCEPT/NEED:** Pain

**NURSING DIAGNOSIS:** Alteration in comfort: pain related to inflammation

**GOAL:** Increased comfort as evidenced by: verbalization, reduced request for pain medication, absence of grimacing

| INTERVENTION | RATIONALE |
|---|---|
| **II. Assess for:** | |
| A. Gastrointestinal assessment to include history and physical exam | A. Needed for data base |
| B. Epigastric pain occurs 45–60 minutes after meals, nocturnally, or in fasting state | B. Pain is related to erosion and inflammation of mucous lining |
| C. Pain is relieved by food, milk, antacids, or vomiting | C. Pain is related to erosion and inflammation of mucous lining |
| D. Pain is described as burning, gnawing, aching, cramping | D. Pain is related to erosion and inflammation of mucous lining |
| E. Epigastric pain and abdominal muscle guarding upon examination | E. Pain is related to erosion and inflammation of mucous lining |
| **III. Administer:** | |
| A. Antacids as ordered | A. Relieves pain |
| B. Antispasmodics as ordered | B. ↓ muscle spasms |
| C. Analgesics as ordered | C. Controls pain |
| **IV. Perform/Provide:** | |
| A. Semi-Fowler's position | A. Promotes comfort |

## V. Teach patient/family:

A. Basic knowledge about disease process

A. Promotes comfort

B. Name of medication, purpose, dosage, time to administer, side effects

B. Insures safe administration

---

**CONCEPT/NEED:** Nutrition

**NURSING DIAGNOSIS:** Alteration in nutrition: less than body requirements related to anorexia

**GOAL:** Adequate nutrition as evidenced by: absence of nausea, eating all meals

## INTERVENTION

## RATIONALE

### II. Assess for:

A. Anorexia, dehydration

A. Compromises nutritional status

B. Nausea and vomiting eructation

B. Compromises nutritional status

C. WT loss, fatigue

C. Compromises nutritional status

D. Nutritional assessment to include 24-hour diet recall, usual eating patterns/history

D. History of inconsistent eating patterns

E. Alcohol, tobacco, aspirin use/abuse

E. Ulcerogenic drugs

F. Complications such as slow, shallow respirations, irritability, disorientation, tremors, tetany

F. Alkalosis from antacid therapy

G. Complications such as muscle flaccidity, weakness, lethargy, cramping

G. Possible potassium deficit in vomiting patients

H. Complications such as weakness, thirst, hypotension, and increased thready pulse

H. Sodium deficit in vomiting patients

I. Complications such as fetid breath, distention, obstipation, nausea, and vomiting

I. S&S of obstruction

J. Barium, swallow and x-ray

J. Reveals ulcerated area in gastric mucosa

K. Gastroscopy

K. Reveals presence of ulcer

L. Gastric analysis

L. Presence of free hydrochloric acid, to differentiate between gastric ulcer and carcinoma of stomach

M. Stool specimen for occult blood

M. Indicates bleeding

## III. Administer:

A. Blood replacement therapy as ordered

A. Replaces blood loss

B. Fluid and electrolytes as ordered

B. Corrects imbalance

C. Antacids as ordered

C. Neutralizes gastric acidity

D. Hydrogen receptor antagonists as ordered

D. Inhibits gastric secretion and promotes healing

E. Anticholinergics as ordered

E. ↓ gastric acid and pepsin secretion

F. Laxatives as ordered

F. Promotes elimination and compensates for lack of roughage

## IV. Perform/Provide:

A. Diet free of strong tea, coffee, cola beverages, alcohol, chocolate, or hot spices

A. Acid-producing or mucosa-irritating substances

B. Restricted use of whole grains, fried eggs, fresh fruits and vegetables, and rich pastries

B. Irritants of intestinal mucosa

C. Small frequent feeding with in-between meal snacks

C. Prevents fasting state and overeating which increases acid secretion

D. Diet of bland, protein foods

D. Buffers gastric acidity, decreases gastric secretion and mobility

E. Unhurried leisurely meal time, chew food slowly

E. ↓ stress and anxiety

F. Nasogastric tube as ordered

F. For excessive nausea and vomiting

## V. Teach patient/family:

A. Maintain regular pattern of small frequent meals

B. Avoid smoking, alcohol, caffeine products, spicy foods, and uncooked fruits and vegetables

C. Avoid stress during mealtime, to eat slowly and chew food well

D. Name of medication, purpose, dosage, time to administer, and side effects

E. Avoid taking more antacid than ordered

F. Avoid taking aspirin and OTC drugs without checking with physician first

G. Identify and eliminate foods that irritate GI system

A. Avoids fasting state and prevents increase acid secretion from overeating

B. Irritates GI tract

C. ↓ gastric secretions

D. Insures safe administration

E. Possible alkalosis from antacid overdose

F. Irritant to GI tract, increases acid production, bleeding

G. Individuals vary in the foods that irritate their system

---

**CONCEPT/NEED:** Anxiety

**NURSING DIAGNOSIS:** Anxiety related to lifestyle

**GOAL:** Decreased anxiety as evidenced by: verbalization, planning lifestyle to reduce stress

### INTERVENTION

II. Assess for:
A. Verbal and nonverbal clues to anxiety
B. Prolonged physical or emotional stress, e.g., chronic illness, divorce, death in family

### RATIONALE

A. Patient may be unable to express anxiety openly
B. Stress increases gastric secretions

C. Personal resources to cope with financial, emotional, and physical stress
(See Psychosocial Assessment, p. 31)

C. Lack of significant other or poor physical health affects response to stress

## III. Administer:
A. Tranquilizers as ordered
B. Sedatives as ordered

A. Relieves anxiety
B. Promotes rest

## IV. Perform/Provide:
A. Comfortable quiet environment
B. Limitation of visitors that upset patient
C. Explanations about equipment, procedures, tests, and personnel
D. Opportunity for expression of fears and questions regarding condition and dietary restrictions
E. Remain with patient during periods of emotional crisis or periods of hematemesis

A. ↓ anxiety

B. Stress increases gastric secretions

C. ↓ anxiety

D. Fosters open communication

E. Reassures patient, ↓ anxiety

## V. Teach patient/family:
A. Avoid stress and situations known to increase stress. A change in workplace may be needed
B. Rest after meals and exercise
C. The relationship between stress and disease process

A. ↓ stress, ↓ gastric secretions, ↓ irritation of mucosa

B. Limits physical and emotional stress
C. ↑ compliance to stress avoidance

# ■ Gastritis

**DEFINITION:** The inflammation of the stomach mucosa caused by ingestion of highly seasoned or infected food, too hot or too cold foods, or chemicals

**CONCEPT/NEED:** Nutrition

**NURSING DIAGNOSIS:** Alteration in nutrition: less than body requirements related to vomiting

**GOAL:** Adequate nutritional intake as evidenced by: absence of anorexia, vomiting, eating all meals

| INTERVENTION | RATIONALE |
|---|---|
| **II. Assess for:** | |
| A. Gastrointestinal history and physical assessment | A. Provides baseline data |
| B. Anorexia | B. Symptoms of gastritis |
| C. Nausea and vomiting, feeling of fullness, hematemesis may be present | C. Lack of stomach emptying |
| D. Nutritional assessment to include history and foods that irritate condition | D. Needed for data base |
| E. Pernicious anemia, thyroiditis, and Addison's disease | E. May precipitate gastritis |
| F. Complete blood count | F. Mild leukocytosis or leukopenia |
| G. Thirsty, restlessness, increased pulse, pallor, diaphoresis, and tarry stools | G. Signs of complications, e.g., shock, hemorrhage, and electrolyte imbalance |
| **III. Administer:** | |
| A. Blood as ordered | A. For treatment of hemorrhage |
| B. Antiemetics as ordered | B. Controls nausea and vomiting |
| C. Anticholinergics as ordered | C. Reduces gastric spasms |
| D. Antacids as ordered | D. Neutralizes acidity |
| E. Sedatives or tranquilizers as ordered | E. ↓ anxiety which decreases anorexia |

F. Supplementary vitamins K, B, C

    F. K to limit bleeding, B and C vitamins to promote healing

G. Intravenous feedings as ordered

    G. Maintains nutrition and hydration when patient is NPO

## IV. Perform/Provide:

A. Comfortable quiet environment

    A. ↓ anxiety, continues to decrease vagal stimulation and gastric secretions

B. Unhurried leisurely meal time

    B. ↓ emotional pressure

C. Diet free of strong tea, coffee, cola beverages, alcohol, chocolate, hot spices

    C. Acid-producing or mucosa-irritating substances

D. Diet free of or limited in whole grains, fried eggs, fresh fruits, vegetables, and rich pastries

    D. Irritates intestinal mucosa

E. Small frequent feedings

    E. Avoids overeating

## V. Teach patient/family:

A. Basic knowledge about disease process to include relationship to diet

    A. ↑ compliance to treatment

B. Name of medication, dosage, time to administer, purpose, and side effects

    B. Insures safe administration

C. Avoid stress during meal time, eat slowly and chew foods well

    C. ↓ gastric secretions

D. Avoid or restrict alcohol, coffee, tobacco, cocoa, spicy foods, uncooked fruits and vegetables, and aspirin

    D. Irritates GI tract

E. Serve several small meals and in-between meal snacks

    E. Prevents fasting state and overeating (overeating stimulates acid secretion)

# ■ Hemorrhoids/Hemorrhoidectomy/ Rectal Fissure and Fistula

**DEFINITION:** Hemorrhoids are internal or external varicose veins in the anal canal caused by pressure on these veins. Hemorrhoidectomy is the surgical excision of these veins. Rectal fissure is an ulceration of the anal canal resulting from the trauma of passing an excessively large stool. Rectal fistula is a sinus tract that extends from the anal canal to the outside of the anus usually as a result of an abscess

**CONCEPT/NEED:** Pain

**NURSING DIAGNOSIS:** Alteration in comfort: pain related to inflammation

**GOAL:** Increased comfort as evidenced by: verbalization, decreased swelling and itching

| INTERVENTION | RATIONALE |
|---|---|
| II. Assess for: | |
| A. Characteristics, location, and extent of pain | A. Aids in effective pain management |
| B. S&S of inflammation/infection | B. Early detection and treatment |
| C. Comfortable proper body alignment | C. Pain control/comfort, avoid supine if possible |
| D. Proper patterns of nutrition/elimination | D. Constipation may lead to development of hemorroids |
| E. Constipation and rectal bleeding | E. Symptoms of cancer |
| F. Pain (severe) on defecation | F. Indicative of anal fissures |
| G. Drainage on undergarments from anorectal area | G. Anal fistulas |
| H. Urinary retention | H. From pain and discomfort of surgical trauma |
| I. Pruritis in anal area | I. Common symptom of hemorrhoidal inflammation |

### III. Administer:
A. Analgesics as ordered
B. Stool softeners as ordered

C. Antibiotics as ordered

A. Pain relief
B. Prevents pain from hard stool against sutures
C. ↑ comfort, ↓ infection

### IV. Perform/Provide:
A. Pillows between knees if lying on side
B. Good oral hygiene
C. Peri-care PRN after bowel movement
D. Precaution/encouragement during first post-operative bowel movement
(See Post-Operative Care, p. 17)
E. Low residue/soft diet as ordered
F. Gelfoam or flotation pads while sitting in chair (not long periods)
G. Sitz baths as ordered

H. Warm compresses as ordered
I. Rectal tube or drain as ordered

A. ↑ comfort, ↓ pain

B. ↑ comfort
C. Prevents infection

D. ↓ pain/discomfort, possible vertigo

E. Constipation avoidance, comfort
F. ↑ comfort, ↓ pain

G. ↑ comfort, ↓ pain and inflammation
H. ↑ comfort
I. Prevents abdominal distention

### V. Teach patient/family:
A. Proper nutrition as ordered

B. Care of incisional area and warm compresses, petroleum gauze pads as ordered
C. Proper peri-care
D. Avoidance of constipation

E. Avoid heavy lifting
F. S&S of all complications

A. Prevents recurrence, ↑ comfort, avoids constipation
B. ↑ comfort, ↓ inflammation

C. Prevents infection
D. Prevents re-injury, promotes comfort
E. Prevents re-injury
F. Early detection and treatment

**CONCEPT/NEED:** Anxiety

**NURSING DIAGNOSIS:** Anxiety related to pain

**GOAL:** Decreased anxiety as evidenced by: verbalization, pulse WNL, ability to sleep at night

| INTERVENTION | RATIONALE |
|---|---|
| **II. Assess for:** | |
| A. Level of knowledge of treatment/condition | A. Information reduces anxiety |
| B. Verbal and nonverbal clues to anxiety (See Pre-Operative Care, p. 13) | B. Patient may not express feelings in usual manner. |
| **III. Administer:** | |
| A. Anti-anxiety medication as ordered | A. Relieves anxiety |
| **IV. Perform/Provide:** | |
| A. Complete information about condition/treatment | A. Aids in pre- and post-operative teaching, relieves anxiety |
| B. Listening environment for patient to verbalize fears/anxiety | B. Enhances communication/relieves anxiety |
| **V. Teach patient/family:** (See Post-Operative Care, p. 17) | |

# ■ Hepatitis

**DEFINITION:** The inflammation of the liver caused by a virus. May be type A, B, or toxic. Type A, known as infectious hepatitis, transmitted by foods or liquids; type B, known as serum hepatitis, transmitted by mucous membrane or breaks in the skin; and toxic, which is the result of administration of drugs that have damaging effects on the liver

**CONCEPT/NEED:** Fluid balance

**NURSING DIAGNOSIS:** Fluid volume deficit related to decreased intake

**GOAL:** Adequate fluid volume as evidenced by: fluid intake of 2–3 L/day

| INTERVENTION | RATIONALE |
|---|---|
| **I. Monitor, describe, record:** | |
| A. I&O q 8 hr | A. Early detection, dehydration, electrolyte imbalance, decreased urinary output, diarrhea |
| B. Body WT, daily at same time, scale, clothing | B. Early detection of ascites or edema in chronic disease, $H_2O$ retention in acute cases |
| **II. Assess for:** | |
| A. Proper fluid intake 3000 ml/day if not NPO | A. Prevents dehydration |
| B. Patterns of fluid intake | B. Knowledge of fluid habits helpful in planning |
| **III. Administer:** | |
| A. Parenteral fluids as ordered | A. Combats dehydration and accompanying electrolyte imbalance |
| B. Alkalis and belladonna as ordered | B. Combats dyspeptic symptoms, do not administer if emesis is problem |
| C. Antiemetics as ordered | C. Controls emesis, aids in restoration of appetite |

**IV. Perform/Provide:**
  A. Good oral hygiene

    A. Prevents complication, discomfort, resultant anorexia

  B. Adequate fluids if not NPO, 3000 ml/day

    B. Prevents complications of dehydration

**V. Teach patient/family:**
  A. Continue fluids as ordered

    A. Promotes healing, convalescence

  B. Avoid alcohol for 1 year

    B. Taxes impaired liver function

---

**CONCEPT/NEED:** Infection

**NURSING DIAGNOSIS:** Potential infection related to inflammation

**GOAL:** Absence of infection as evidenced by: temperature WNL, serum bilirubin WNL

## INTERVENTION

**I. Monitor, describe, record:**
  A. TPR, BP q 4 hr and PRN

**II. Assess for:**
  A. S&S of inflammatory complications, e.g., anorexia, nausea, vomiting, headache, respiratory infection, aches, pains, malaise, fever, jaundice is late sign, clay-colored stools

  B. Potential problem for patient to contract additional infection

  C. Adequate precautions/isolation measures for viral types

## RATIONALE

A. Early detection of complications of hepatic inflammation

A. Early detection and treatment

B. Good hygiene, skin care, and safety contributes to reduction of infection. Body's defense compromised

C. For type A, gown and gloves; enteric precautions for serum; needle precautions. Home or hospital isolation depending on severity, to reduce potential for transmission

D. Level of knowledge of patient about condition and treatment

E. Serum bilirubin and SGOT

D. Proper knowledge encourages cooperation with treatment

E. Increased in hepatitis

## III. Administer:
A. Antipyretics as ordered
B. Antihistamines as ordered
C. Antibiotics as ordered

A. Fever control
B. Relieves pruritis from jaundice
C. For subsequent secondary infection

## IV. Perform/Provide:
A. Complete information about disease/treatment
B. Isolation and precautions as indicated
C. Skin care as indicated with sponge baths
D. Instructions for proper handwashing/hygiene
E. Emotional support

F. Diversional activities, e.g., TV, radio, books, etc.
G. Frequent visits to patient's room/home as indicated

A. Encourages cooperation, ↓ anxiety
B. Prevents transmission

C. Infection prevention, and relief of pruritis
D. Infection control, prevention of transmission
E. Prevents depression from isolation
F. ↓ psychological complications of isolation
G. ↓ psychological complications of isolation

## V. Teach patient/family:
A. Visit patient frequently.
B. Proper precautions (isolation)
C. S&S of complications
D. Importance of not donating blood
E. Importance of avoiding contact with patients with URIs or other infections
F. Importance of follow-up exams
G. Home health care is available
H. Injections of gamma globulin for infections might be ordered

A. Relieves loneliness of isolation
B. Prevents transmission
C. Early detection/treatment
D. Prevents transmission
E. Body's resistance to infection is compromised
F. Early detection and treatment of complications
G. Provides assistance, emotional support, education
H. As prophylactic for transmission prevention

**CONCEPT/NEED:** Pain/Rest

**NURSING DIAGNOSIS:** Alteration in comfort: pain related to fatigue

**GOAL:** Increased comfort as evidenced by: verbalization, absence of grimacing, reduced request for pain medication

| INTERVENTION | RATIONALE |
|---|---|
| **II. Assess for:** | |
| A. Patterns of sleep/rest | A. Early detection of complications of fatigue |
| B. Characteristics, location, and extent of pain | B. Aids in proper effective pain management/comfort |
| C. Level of knowledge of patient about condition/treatment | C. Encourages compliance with activity restrictions |
| D. S&S of fatigue | D. Body's resistance is compromised |
| E. S&S of complications of immobility | E. Prevents complications |
| **III. Administer:** | |
| A. Analgesics as ordered | A. Pain relief |
| B. Sedatives as ordered | B. Promotes/induces sleep/rest |
| **IV. Perform/Provide:** | |
| A. Proper pain assessment | A. Effective pain management |
| B. Limited activity program as ordered | B. Prevents complications of immobility, fatigue |
| C. Bedrest as ordered (2–3 weeks) | C. Prevents fatigue |
| D. Complete information on condition/treatment | D. Enhances cooperation, prevents complications of fatigue |
| E. Proper body alignment | E. ↑ comfort/healing |
| F. Tight linens, daily bath | F. ↑ comfort |
| G. Quiet environment | G. Prevents fatigue and promotes rest/sleep |
| **V. Teach patient/family:** | |
| A. Limit activity | A. Prevents complication of fatigue |
| B. Obtain adequate sleep/rest | B. Prevents complication of fatigue |
| C. Avoid strenuous or contact sports | C. Prevents fatigue, avoids complication of injury |

**CONCEPT/NEED:** Skin integrity

**NURSING DIAGNOSIS:** Impairment of skin integrity related to excretions on skin

**GOAL:** Absence of skin breakdown as evidenced by: lack of pruritis, absence of itching

## INTERVENTION

II. **Assess for:**
   A. Excessive pruritis
   B. Verbal, nonverbal clues to decreased self-image
   C. Jaundice, skin and sclera
   D. Level of knowledge about condition

III. **Administer:**
   A. Antihistamines as ordered
   B. Special baths as ordered (baking soda)
   C. Lotions as ordered

IV. **Perform/Provide:**
   A. Listening environment for patient to verbalize fears/anxiety/concern
   B. Complete information about condition/treatment/outcome
   C. Proper skin care as ordered

V. **Teach patient/family:**
   A. Jaundiced sclera and skin will subside with recovery
   B. Pruritis will subside with jaundice

## RATIONALE

A. Complication of jaundice
B. Patient may not express feelings in usual manner
C. Late sign of hepatitis
D. Information reduces anxiety and fear


A. Relieves pruritis
B. Relieves pruritis

C. Relieves pruritis


A. Promotes communication


B. Enhances cooperation, relieves fear/anxiety
C. Relief of pruritis, infection prevention


A. Relieves anxiety/fear of altered self-image
B. Relieves anxiety/fear of altered self-image

# ■ Hernia/Herniorrhaphy

**DEFINITION:** A protrusion of a part of the viscera through a congenital or acquired weakness in the abdominal wall. May be direct or indirect and occur in the femoral, inguinal, umbilical, or incisional areas. Herniorrhaphy is the surgical repair of a hernia

**CONCEPT/NEED:** Pain

**NURSING DIAGNOSIS:** Alteration in comfort: pain related to trauma

**GOAL:** Increased comfort as evidenced by: verbalization, reduced request for pain medication, lack of grimacing

| INTERVENTION | RATIONALE |
|---|---|
| **II. Assess for:** | |
| A. Characteristics, location, and extent of pain | A. Necessary for effective pain control |
| B. Verbal and nonverbal clues to discomfort | B. Patient may have difficulty verbalizing discomfort |
| C. Pre-operative history | C. Diseases of respiratory system and chronic cough will cause increased intra-abdominal pressure, incision and repair will be compromised |
| D. Post-operative respiratory infection | D. Diseases of respiratory system and chronic cough will cause increased intra-abdominal pressure, incision and repair will be compromised |
| E. Urinary retention | E. ↑ comfort, ↓ pain |
| F. Constipation | F. Intra-abdominal pressure |
| G. Excessive inguinal edema (See Post-Operative Care, p. 17) | G. ↓ pain, ↑ comfort, urinary retention |
| **III. Administer:** | |
| A. Analgesics as ordered | A. Pain relief/control |
| B. Mild catharactics | B. Prevents constipation |

## IV. Perform/Provide:
A. Pain assessment

A. Effective pain management

B. Comprehensive pre-operative history
(See Pre/Post-Operative Care, p. 13, p. 17)

B. Detects respiratory problems before repair

C. NG or rectal tube

C. Abdominal distention is undesirable

D. Ice packs to scrotum as ordered

D. Pain relief

E. Scrotal support as ordered (or elevate as ordered)

E. ↑ comfort, ↓ pain

## V. Teach patient/family:
A. Avoid constipation

A. Increased intra-abdominal pressure, ↓ pain/discomfort, ↑ safety

---

**CONCEPT/NEED:** Anxiety

**NURSING DIAGNOSIS:** Anxiety related to surgery

**GOAL:** Anxiety reduced as evidenced by: verbalization, pulse WNL, ability to sleep at night

## INTERVENTION

## RATIONALE

## II. Assess for:
A. Verbal and nonverbal clues to anxiety

A. Patient may have difficulty expressing feelings in usual manner

B. Patient's level of knowledge about procedure/treatment

B. Information and understanding reduces anxiety

## III. Administer:
A. Anti-anxiety drugs as ordered

A. Anxiety relief

## IV. Perform/Provide:
A. Complete information about procedure/condition

A. Anxiety relief

B. Need to support or splint incision when coughing

B. Prevents re-injury

C. Environmental safety
(See  Pre/Post-Operative
Care, p. 13, p. 17

C. Avoids falls or slips

## V. Teach patient/family:
A. Stand straight
B. Not to lift heavy objects
C. Not to exercise strenuously
D. Patient may need to change
occupation

A. Avoids posture problem
B. May cause re-injury
C. May cause re-injury
D. Prevents re-injury

# ■ Intestinal Obstruction

**DEFINITION:** An impairment of the normal flow of intestinal contents by a partial or complete blockage caused by mechanical, vascular, or nervous conditions

**CONCEPT/NEED:** Pain

**NURSING DIAGNOSIS:** Alteration in comfort: pain related to obstruction

**GOAL:** Increased comfort as evidenced by: verbalization, reduced request for pain medications

| INTERVENTION | RATIONALE |
|---|---|
| **II. Assess for:** | |
| A. Characteristics, location, and extent of pain | A. Large bowel obstruction, mild abdominal pain and discomfort, small bowel obstruction, severe cramping, abdominal pain |
| B. Verbal and nonverbal clues to discomfort | B. Vomiting and pain emotionally drain patient |
| C. Clues to respiratory distress | C. Intestinal distention may interfere with respiration |
| D. Discomfort related to urinary retention | D. Due to distention pressure on bladder |
| **III. Administer:** | |
| A. Avoid opiates, give analgesics as ordered | A. Pain relief |
| B. Anti-anxiety drugs as ordered | B. ↓ anxiety |
| C. Anti-emetics as ordered | C. ↓ nausea/vomiting |
| **IV. Perform/Provide:** | |
| A. Assistance in turning in bed | A. ↑ comfort |
| B. Emotional support | B. Alleviates anxiety, promotes comfort |

| | |
|---|---|
| C. Rectal tube as ordered | C. Relieves distention |
| D. Enemas or colonic irrigations as ordered | D. Relieves distention |
| E. Meticulous skin and mouth care | E. ↑ comfort |
| F. Immediate removal of vomitus | F. Usually foul odor, causes nausea and discomfort |
| G. Fowler's position | G. For respiratory distress |
| H. Proper body alignment | H. ↑ comfort |
| I. Quiet atmosphere | I. ↑ comfort |

**V. Teach patient/family:**

| | |
|---|---|
| A. Breathe through nose | A. Swallowing air increases distention |
| B. About impending surgery if indicated or other procedure | B. Prevents undue anxiety, relief of pain |

---

**CONCEPT/NEED:** Fluid balance

**NURSING DIAGNOSIS:** Fluid volume deficit related to vomiting

**GOAL:** Adequate fluid volume as evidenced by: absence of vomiting, weight maintenance, electrolytes WNL

## INTERVENTION

## RATIONALE

**I. Monitor, describe, record:**

| | |
|---|---|
| A. TPR, BP q 4 hr | A. Early detection of complications |
| B. I&O q 8 hr | B. Assess for fluid imbalance |
| C. Electrolytes | C. Imbalance due to vomiting |

**III. Administer:**

| | |
|---|---|
| A. Parenteral fluids as ordered | A. Combats dehydration, electrolyte imbalance |
| B. Hyperalimentation as ordered | B. For pre-operative patients who are in severe nutritional deficit |
| C. Antiemetics as ordered | C. ↓ vomiting |

**IV. Perform/Provide:**

| | |
|---|---|
| A. Extensive nutrition/elimination assessment | A. Necessary for proper diagnosis |

B. Adequate fluids if indicated 3000 ml/day

C. Good oral care

D. Bowel sounds q 2 hr

E. Girth of abdomen q 4 hr

B. Combats complications of dehydration

C. Fecal vomitus

D. High pitched, peristaltic rushes are diagnostic

E. Increasing distention indicated

## V. Teach patient/family:

A. Proper nutrition

B. Chew food completely and eat slowly

C. Maintain adequate fluid intake if possible

D. S&S of complications

A. Helps with compliance

B. Aids in digestion

C. Avoids constipation

D. Early detection and treatment

# ■ Pancreatitis

**DEFINITION:** An inflammatory disease of the pancreas thought to result from the use of alcohol, tumors, trauma, or biliary tract disease. May be acute or chronic and progressive

**CONCEPT/NEED:** Fluid balance

**NURSING DIAGNOSIS:** Fluid volume deficit related to vomiting

**GOAL:** Adequate fluid intake as evidenced by: normal electrolyte levels, absence of vomiting, intake of 2–3 L/day

| INTERVENTION | RATIONALE |
|---|---|
| **I. Monitor, describe, record:** | |
| A. TPR, BP q 4 hr as needed | A. Early detection and treatment of complications, shock, and infections |
| B. I&O q 8 hr | B. Early detection of ascites, dehydration |
| **II. Assess for:** | |
| A. Extent of nausea and vomiting | A. Early detection of fluid and electrolyte imbalance |
| B. Signs of shock | B. Hypovolemia-ascites, hemorrhage due to auto-digestion of pancreas |
| C. Signs of dehydration | C. Occurs from nausea/vomiting |
| D. Proper nutrition and fluid intake | D. May appear malnourished and dehydrated (chronic) |
| E. S&S of diabetes mellitus | E. Present if cells of Islet of Langerhans are affected |
| F. Excessive intake or addiction to alcohol | F. Abuse is related to this condition |
| G. WBC/blood studies | G. Elevated serum amylase-lipase, usually elevated WBC |
| H. Urine for sugar q 2 hr | H. Signs of diabetes/glycosuria |
| I. Abdominal girth q 4 hr | I. Early detection of ascites, dehydration |

J. Bowel sounds q 2 hr      J. Assess for bowel obstruction

K. Serum glucose      K. Transient hyperglycemia

L. Electrolytes      L. Imbalance related to dehydration

M. Liver function studies      M. May be elevated

N. Blood calcium level      N. Hypocalcemia may result

## III. Administer:

A. Parenteral fluids as ordered      A. Corrects deficit volume of electrolyte

B. Anticholinergics as ordered      B. ↓ pancreatic secretion

C. Aprotinin as ordered      C. Inhibits trypsin, inactivates kallikrein

D. Antibiotics as ordered      D. Infection is seen frequently

E. Corticosteroids as ordered      E. For severe fulminating pancreatitis

F. O$_2$ and IPPB as ordered      F. Prevents respiratory complications

G. Insulin as ordered      G. For pancreas failure

## IV. Perform/Provide:

A. Information on nutrition and fluid intake if appropriate      A. Prevents complication of dehydration and malnutrition in post-acute phase

B. NPO as ordered      B. Food stimulates pancreatic secretion

C. NG suctioning as ordered      C. ↓ pancreatic secretion

D. Avoidance of alcohol, spices, and coffee      D. Aggravates condition

E. How to test urine      E. Glycosuria

F. Insulin administration as ordered      F. Avoids dangerous complications

G. S&S of complications      G. Early detection/treatment

H. Availability of alcoholic counseling if applicable      H. Treats alcoholism

I. Bedrest as ordered      I. Avoids complications of fatigue

J. CVP as ordered      J. Monitors fluid volume

---

**CONCEPT/NEED:** Pain

**NURSING DIAGNOSIS:** Alteration in comfort: pain related to inflammation

**GOAL:** Increased comfort as evidenced by: verbalization, absence of grimacing, reduced request in pain medication

| INTERVENTION | RATIONALE |
|---|---|
| **II. Assess for:** | |
| A. Verbal and nonverbal clues to discomfort | A. Patient may not express feelings in usual manner |
| B. Characteristics, location, and extent of pain | B. Aids in effective pain management |
| C. Patient's level of knowledge about condition | C. Information may relieve anxiety |
| D. Proper body alignment | D. ↑ comfort, ↑ ventilation |
| **III. Administer:** | |
| A. Anti-anxiety drugs as ordered | A. ↓ anxiety |
| B. Anticholinergics as ordered | B. ↓ pancreatic secretions |
| C. Analgesic as ordered | C. ↓ pain |
| **IV. Perform/Provide:** | |
| A. Complete information on condition/treatment | A. Anxiety relief |
| B. Accurate pain assessment | B. Effective pain management |
| C. Listening environment for patient to verbalize feelings | C. Anxiety reduction through communication |
| D. Proper body alignment | D. ↑ comfort |
| E. Fowler's position | E. ↓ discomfort from pressure on diaphragm from distended abdomen, comfort/ventilation |
| F. Bedrest as ordered | A. ↓ metabolic rate, pancreatic secretions, spasms, pain |
| G. Accurate pain assessment | B. Pain control |
| **V. Teach patient/family:** | |
| A. Avoid stress at meal time | A. Aids in proper digestion |

# ■ Total Parenteral Nutrition/ Hyperalimentation

**DEFINITION:** Total nutritional needs supplied by catheter inserted into the subclavian vein. Includes nutrients, water, and electrolytes needed to maintain a positive nitrogen balance.

## INTERVENTION

### I. Monitor, describe, record:
A. VS q 4 hr
B. I&O q 8 hr
C. WT QD
D. Serum electrolytes
E. Flow rate q 1 hr
F. Urine for glucose q 8 hr, specific gravity decrease
G. Blood glucose, CBC

### II. Assess for:
A. Dehydration to include WT loss, skin turgor, thirst
B. Catheter dressing for looseness, drainage, wetness
C. Activity and movement and ROM in bed
D. Content of solution, contamination, expiration
E. Tissue at insertion site for swelling, pain
F. Tube patency
G. Signs of respiratory difficulty, dyspnea
H. Signs of hyperglycemia to include lethargy, twitching
I. Signs of hypoglycemia to include muscle weakness, vertigo, pallor
J. Allergy to solution, rash, chills

### III. Administer:
A. TPN solution per order with appropriate administration set, never add drugs to solution. Never administer blood or blood products or drugs through TPN catheter

### IV. Perform/Provide:
A. Change dressing QD and PRN using aseptic technique, patient in low Fowler's position
B. Change tubing and filter, patient to perform Valsalva maneuver
C. Change of position q 2–4 hr
D. Skin care over bony prominences

E. Active and passive ROM
F. Regulated administration of solution using an infusion pump
G. Opportunity to express feelings
H. Removal of catheter in safe manner

## V. Teach patient family:
A. Protection of site, not to pull on catheter
B. Why I&O is important to record
C. Importance of ambulation, movement
D. Report rash, chills, pain, change in breathing, fatigue

# ■ Ulcerative Colitis/ Regional Enteritis

**DEFINITION:** Ulcerative colitis is the inflammation of the mucosa and submucosa of the colon and rectum resulting in diarrhea with blood and mucus, fever, vomiting, and abdominal cramping, and weight loss

**CONCEPT/NEED:** Nutrition

| INTERVENTION | RATIONALE |
|---|---|
| **I. Monitor, describe, record:** | |
| A. I&O q 8 hr | A. Early detection of fluid imbalance |
| B. Daily body WT with same scale, clothes, time | B. WT loss from dehydration/malnutrition |
| **II. Assess for:** | |
| A. History of GI disease | A. Needed for data base |
| B. Patterns of nutrition | B. Certain types of foods may irritate bowel (spices, milk) |
| C. Proper fluid intake 3000 ml/day | C. Prevents dehydration |
| **III. Administer:** | |
| A. Antiemetics as ordered | A. Combats nausea/vomiting |
| B. High protein, low residue, high carbohydrate | B. Aids in digestion |
| C. TPN as ordered | C. In severely debilitated patients |
| D. NPO as ordered | D. May be needed to rest bowel |
| E. Iron dextran | E. Combats anemia |
| **IV. Perform/Provide:** | |
| A. Good oral hygiene | A. Aids appetite |
| B. Fluids 3000 ml/day | B. Prevents dehydration |
| **V. Teach patient/family:** | |
| A. Eat slowly/completely chew food | A. Aids digestion |
| B. Avoid stressful meal times | B. Aids appetite |
| C. Proper nutrition | C. Assists in compliance |

D. Eat small frequent meals
E. Avoid dairy products, spicy foods, hot/cold foods

D. Aids appetite
E. Hard to digest

---

**CONCEPT/NEED:** Skin integrity

**NURSING DIAGNOSIS:** Impairment of skin integrity related to excretions on skin

**GOAL:** Skin integrity as evidenced by: absence of redness around anus

## INTERVENTION

**I. Monitor, describe, record:**
   A. TPR, BP q 4 hr

**II. Assess for:**
   A. S&S of infection
   B. Bowel sounds q 4 hr

**III. Administer:**
   A. Steroid therapy as ordered
   B. Antibiotics as ordered
   C. Antidiarrheals
   D. Anticholinergics as ordered

**IV. Perform/Provide:**
   A. Abdominal girth q shift
   B. Hemoccult of stool
   C. Privacy, soft tissue, room deodorizer
   D. Keep bedpan within easy reach and empty and return quickly

**V. Teach patient/family:**
   A. Good peri-care
   B. Use ointments for anorectal irritation
   C. Avoid foods which increase peristalsis or diarrhea

## RATIONALE

A. Early detection of inflammation/ infection

A. Early detection
B. Detects obstruction

A. Anti-inflammatory
B. Combats infection
C. Combats diarrhea
D. ↓ motility

A. Abdominal distention
B. Occult blood
C. Comforts during elimination

D. ↑ comfort

A. Avoidance of infection
B. ↑ comfort, inflammation prevention
C. ↓ chance for irritation

**CONCEPT/NEED:** Pain

**NURSING DIAGNOSIS:** Alteration in comfort: pain related to inflammation

**GOAL:** Increased comfort as evidenced by: verbalization, absence of grimacing

| INTERVENTION | RATIONALE |
|---|---|
| **II. Assess for:** | |
| A. Characteristic, location, and extent of pain | A. Aids in proper pain management |
| B. Verbal, nonverbal clues to anxiety/fear | B. Patient may be unable to express feelings in usual manner |
| C. Patterns of activity/rest | C. For planning |
| **III. Administer:** | |
| A. Analgesics as ordered | A. Pain relief, ↑ comfort |
| B. Tranquilizers as ordered | B. Combats anxiety |
| C. Antispasmodics as ordered | C. Comfort, relief of spasms, cramps |
| **IV. Perform/Provide:** | |
| A. Quiet, listening environment for patient to verbalize feelings | A. ↓ anxiety |
| B. Backrubs | B. Provides relaxation |
| C. Muscle relaxation techniques | C. Combats anxiety |
| D. Restrict visitors if necessary | D. Stress avoidance |
| **V. Teach patient/family:** | |
| A. Stress avoidance | A. Stress aggravates and precipitates condition |
| B. Avoid fatigue | B. Fatigue aggravates condition |
| C. About availability of emotional counseling | C. Emotional stress is related to disease |

# RENAL SYSTEM STANDARDS

- Renal System Assessment
- Chronic Renal Failure (Uremia)
- Cystitis
- Glomerulonephritis/Pyelonephritis
- Intravenous Therapy
- Nephrectomy/Nephrostomy
- Renal Calculi/Urolithiasis
- Urinary Catheter

# ■ Renal System Assessment

**DEFINITION:** The collection of a data base concerning the renal system and its functional capabilities to be used in identifying nursing problems related to fluid-electrolyte and acid-base balance

## INTERVENTION

I. **Interview and investigate for and record past history:**
   A. Previous renal conditions such as calculi, pyelonephritis, cystitis, hypertension
   B. Previous operations, injury, pregnancy, or other chronic medical conditions related to kidneys
   C. Allergies and immunizations
   D. Pain in kidney or urinary bladder area
   E. Urinary infections, incontinence, retention, dribbling, urgency, frequency, burning
   F. Special diet to prevent calculi formation
   G. Usual pattern of urine elimination and if patient gets up at night to void (frequency, what times during day)
   H. Usual characteristics of urine (amount, color, odor, sedimentation, hematuria, polyuria, oliguria)
   I. Edema, distention, fever, chills, bruising, restlessness, insomnia, itching skin
   J. Sexually transmitted diseases
   K. Medications taken for kidney or urinary conditions and response (prescription and OTC)
   L. Past cystoscopy, KUB, IVP, scans, urinalysis, BUN, creatinine, PSP, creatinine clearance, or other tests and results
   M. Usual type and amount of fluid intake/output for 24 hr
   N. Dryness of mucous membranes, skin, lips, poor skin turgor
   O. Past ABGs or serum electrolytes and results
   P. Symptoms of increased or decreased potassium, sodium, calcium

II. **Interview and investigate for and record present history:**
   A. Chief complaint
   B. Onset and length of illness
   C. Principal S&S
   D. Knowledge of disease, procedures, and planned therapy
   E. Urinary drainage devices and any other treatments

F. Results of KUB, CBC, urinalysis and culture, ABGs electrolytes, BUN, IVP, renal clearance tests, scans

G. Medications being taken for urinary, renal problems

## III. Inspection/Observation for:

A. I&O q 8 hr

B. Presence of dehydration to include thirst, WT loss, poor skin turgor, dry skin and mucous membranes, oliguria, confusion

C. Presence of edema in ankles, feet, sacrum, rapid weight gain, distention (abdominal)

D. Characteristics of urinary output

E. Indwelling catheter patency and position of bag

F. Cleanliness of meatal area around catheter

G. Dysuria, hematuria, oliguria, polyuria, retention, incontinence, frequency, urgency, burning, dribbling

H. Fever, chills, pain in kidney area and if radiating, fatigue, restlessness, itching of skin, insomnia

I. Elevated BP, neck vein distention or collapse, nausea, confusion, muscle weakness, numbness, tingling, muscle cramps and twitching, cardiac arrhythmias, rapid, deep breathing or slow shallow breathing, headache, lethargy and other S&S of fluid-electrolyte and acid-base imbalance.

J. IV fluid and electrolyte replacement

K. Excessive vomiting, diarrhea, NG tube drainage, dyspnea

L. Daily WT on same scale, at same time and with same clothing

M. Surgical dressings for drainage, reinforcement if surgery done

N. Changes in self-image associated with indwelling catheter

## IV. Palpation for:

A. Size and movability of kidneys

B. Pain in kidney area

C. Bladder distention

# ■ Chronic Renal Failure (Uremia)

**DEFINITION:** A group of symptoms resulting from a gradual deterioration of kidney function which can be caused by hypertension, glomerulonephritis, or chronic pyelonephritis

**CONCEPT/NEED:** Fluid/Electrolyte balance

**NURSING DIAGNOSIS:** Fluid volume excess related to decreased output

**GOAL:** Adequate fluid volume as evidenced by: absence of edema, BP WNL

| INTERVENTION | RATIONALE |
|---|---|
| **I. Monitor, describe, record:** | |
| A. I&O character of urine q 1–8 hr as needed | A. Total intake should not exceed previous day's urinary output plus 600–800 ml |
| B. WT QD same time, scale, clothing | B. Should not vary more than 1 lb/day |
| **II. Assess:** | |
| A. Renal system assessment for history and physical examination | A. Needed for data base |
| B. Increased respiration, flaccid paralysis, arrhythmias, nausea, diarrhea | B. S&S of hyperkalemia, protein catabolism releases intercellular potassium |
| C. Palpitations, weak irregular pulse, dizziness, faintness | C. S&S of hypokalemia due to overtreatment of hyperkalemia |
| D. Weight gain, edema, dry flushed skin, weak pulse, tachycardia, fever, tremors | D. S&S of hypernatremia due to kidney's ability to excrete sodium |
| E. Decreased BP, abdominal cramps, headache, weakness, faintness | E. S&S of hyponatremia due to overtreatment of hypernatremia |
| F. Convulsions, tetany, muscle spasms, irregular pulse | F. S&S of hypocalcemia due to decreased calcium absorption from intestine |

G. Pathological fractures, nausea and vomiting, deep bone pain, irregular pulse

H. Oliguria to anuria

I. Pitting edema and/or rapid WT gain, peri-orbital edema

J. Blood chemistries to include BUN, serum creatinine, uric acid, chloride, electrolytes, pH

K. Renal function studies

L. Renal dilution and concentration tests

M. Urine culture

N. Urinalysis

O. IVP or renal arteriography

P. Renography

G. S&S of hypercalcemia due to mobilization of calcium from bones

H. Indicates renal shutdown

I. Increased fluid retention. Kidneys unable to excrete $H_2O$

J. Increased BUN, creatinine, uric acid and chloride: hyponatremia, hypocalcemia, hyperkalemia, hypermagnesemia and hyperphosphatemia, decreased pH, sodium bicarbonate

K. Decreased creatinine, phenosulfophthalein excretion in urine

L. Decreased ability to concentrate urine

M. Reveals organisms if present

N. Gross and microscopic hematuria, decreased specific gravity, sodium content

O. Decreased kidney function and perfusion

P. Decreased uptake and secretion of the radioisotope by each kidney

## III. Administer:

A. Peritoneal dialysis or hemodialysis as ordered

B. Diuretics as ordered

C. Exchange resins as ordered

D. Chelating agents as ordered

E. Adrenergic drugs as ordered

F. Antibiotic as ordered

G. Calcium carbonate as ordered. Vitamin D supplement

H. Parenteral fluids with electrolytes as ordered

I. Phosphate binders

A. Removes toxic wastes and helps correct fluid and electrolyte balance

B. ↓ fluid overload

C. Promotes excretion of excess electrolytes

D. Binds toxic metals

E. ↑ renal blood flow

F. Prevents and limits infection

G. For hypocalcemia

H. If electrolytes are decreased

I. ↓ phosphate in blood

## IV. Perform/Provide:

A. Ice chips if fluid is being restricted

B. Restrict fluid intake as determined by urinary losses

C. Restrict sodium and potassium as necessary

A. Helps extend limited fluid

B. Intake should not exceed previous day's output plus 600–800 ml

C. Prevents hypernatremia and hyperkalemia

## V. Teach patient/family:

A. Amount of fluid daily allowed in the diet

B. Purpose of restricted intake

C. Measure output

D. Observe character of urine

E. Report decreased or absent urination, edema of extremities or eyes

F. How to keep I&O record including daily weight

G. Avoid cold cuts, cured meats, milk and dairy products, olives, beans, beets, pickles, soups, and meat tenderizers

H. Avoid oranges, bananas, dried fruits, melons, beans, peas and green leafy vegetables, milk

I. Use herbs and spices

J. Name of medication, purpose, time to administer, dosage, and side effects

A. ↑ compliance

B. ↑ compliance

C. Includes urine and emesis

D. For color, consistency

E. Indicates complications

F. ↑ compliance

G. High in sodium

H. High in potassium

I. Season food without salt

J. Insures safe administration

---

**CONCEPT/NEED:** Nutrition

**NURSING DIAGNOSIS:** Alteration in nutrition: less than body requirements related to anorexia

**GOAL:** Adequate nutritional intake as evidenced by: absence of anorexia, eating protein-restricted diet

| INTERVENTION | RATIONALE |
|---|---|

**I. Monitor, describe, record:**

A. WT QD with same clothing, scale, time of day     A. Insures accurate weight

**II. Assess for:**

A. Anorexia, nausea, vomiting, and weight loss     A. May indicate reduced nutrition

B. Fruity breath     B. ↑ ketone bodies

C. Bitter metallic taste in mouth     C. Due to levels of nitrogenous waste

D. Ulcerations of mouth     D. May cause decrease in food intake

E. BUN, creatine clearance results     E. Indicates build-up of waste

**III. Administer:**

A. Antacids as ordered     A. For control of gastric acid

B. Antiemetics as ordered     B. For control of nausea

C. Iron, calcium, and vitamin supplements as ordered     C. For needed nutrients

**IV. Perform/Provide:**

A. Low sodium, low protein, high carbohydrate, high fat, low potassium diet as ordered     A. ↓ fluid retention

B. Increase protein intake only if on dialysis     B. End products will raise protein in blood

C. Frequent oral hygiene     C. For halitosis

D. Hard candies     D. ↑ carbohydrate content

E. Hyperalimentation as ordered     E. If diet cannot be tolerated by mouth

F. Protein restriction if creatinine clearance is below 10 ml/min and BUN is above 100 mg/10 ml and acidosis develops     F. Serum albumin will fall if protein restriction is too severe

G. Caloric intake 40 cal/kg of ideal body WT     G. Maintains ideal body weight

H. Intake of high quality protein, e.g., eggs, poultry, and fish     H. Avoids proteins that do not contain all the essential amino acids

I. Increase amount of concentrated carbohydrates and fats, e.g, candies, marshmallows, sugar, jellies, and salt-free margarine

I. Maintains caloric intake while decreasing protein intake

## V. Teach patient/family:
A. Maintain diet as ordered

A. Maintains nutrition within restrictions

B. Carefully read all labels on food

B. Many foods contain sodium and potassium

C. Avoid excessive protein intake

C. Increases protein in blood

---

**CONCEPT/NEED:** Skin integrity

**NURSING DIAGNOSIS:** Impairment of skin integrity related to pruritis/stomatitis

**GOAL:** Skin integrity as evidenced by: absence of pruritis, absence of stomatitis

## INTERVENTION

## RATIONALE

### II. Assess for:
A. Usual hygiene patterns

A. Needed for data base

B. Pruritis

B. Due to irritation from evaporated uremic frost

C. Uremic frost on skin

C. From high level of waste in system

D. Halitosis

D. Ammonia odor

E. Ulcerations of mouth

E. Result of uremia

F. Dry scaly skin

F. Result of uremic dermatitis

G. Yellow-tan or bronze tone skin coloring

G. Retention of pigments normally excreted by kidney

H. Brittle hair and nails

H. Retention of waste products

I. Decreased perspiration

I. Smaller sweat glands

### IV. Perform/Provide:
A. Skin care q 4 hr with lanolin-based lotion

A. Prevents skin drying and cracking

| B. Perineal care BID and PRN | B. Prevents UTI |
| C. Aseptic techniques when caring for urinary catheters, hyperalimentation, catheters, and dressings | C. (See Urinary Catheters and Hyperalimentation, p. 262, p. 297) |
| D. Avoid use of soap | D. Dries the skin |

**V. Teach patient/family:**

| A. Importance of good handwashing | A. Avoids spread of organisms |
| B. Apply lanolin-based lotion | B. Prevents skin drying and cracking |

---

**CONCEPT/NEED:** Transport/Circulation

**NURSING DIAGNOSIS:** Alteration in tissue perfusion related to blood loss

**GOAL:** Adequate tissue perfusion as evidenced by: normal VS

**INTERVENTION**

**RATIONALE**

**I. Monitor, describe, record:**

| A. BP q 4 hr and PRN, pulse q 4 hr and PRN | A. Reduced in hemorrhage |

**II. Assess:**

| A. Cardiovascular assessment to include history and physical examination | A. Needed for data base |
| B. Shortness of breath, breath sounds | B. Related to fluid loss |
| C. Anemia | C. From azotemia |
| D. Ventricular hypertrophy | D. Adaptation to decreased $O_2$ carrying ability |
| E. Pericarditis | E. From increased nitrogenous wastes in blood |
| F. Cardiac tamponade | F. Complication of pericarditis |
| G. Bleeding tendency | G. Related to defective platelets |
| H. Hgb and Hct | H. Decreased due to anemia |

I. CBC

J. Platelet count and platelet aggregation

I. Decreased in maturity and quality of erythrocytes

J. Normal platelet count decreases aggregation

## III. Administer:
A. Packed blood cells as ordered
(See Blood/Blood Products, Transfusion, p. 160)

A. For anemia

## IV. Perform/Provide:
A. Soft tooth brushes
B. Assist patient to turn, cough and deep breathe q 4 hr

A. ↓ or prevents bleeding
B. Raises sputum, ↑ lung expansion

## V. Teach patient/family:
A. Avoid aspirin and OTC drugs
B. Maintain dietary limitations of sodium and potassium

A. May increase bleeding tendencies

B. Increase in sodium and potassium cause arrhythmias

---

**CONCEPT/NEED:** Orientation

**NURSING DIAGNOSIS:** Sensory perception alteration related to decreasing orientation

**GOAL:** Adequate sensory perception as evidenced by: oriented ×3, absence of hallucinations/delusions

## INTERVENTION

## RATIONALE

II. **Assess for:**
A. Orientation q 4 hr
B. Delusions and hallucinations
C. Stupor, convulsions, and coma
D. Seizure activity
E. Muscular twitching and numbness

A. Needed for data base
B. Caused by uremia
C. Caused by uremia

D. ↑ amonia level
E. Peripheral neuropathy occurs

### III. Administer:
| | |
|---|---|
| A. Anticonvulsants as ordered | A. Raises seizure threshold |
| B. Sedatives as ordered | B. Promotes rest, raises seizure threshold |

### IV. Perform/Provide:
| | |
|---|---|
| A. Airway, side rails up and bed in low position | A. Seizure precautions |

### V. Teach patient/family:
| | |
|---|---|
| A. Change in orientation is due to disease process | A. ↓ anxiety |

---

**CONCEPT/NEED:** Sexuality

**NURSING DIAGNOSIS:** Sexual dysfunction related to decreased libido

**GOAL:** Sexual function as evidenced by: menstrual regularity, absence of impotence

## INTERVENTION

## RATIONALE

### II. Assess for:
| | |
|---|---|
| A. Delayed puberty in children | A. Endocrine gland function impaired due to uremia |
| B. Decreased libido, impotency, decreased sperm count and infertility, amenorrhea | B. Impaired due to uremia |
| C. Depression, anxiety, or altered self-image | C. Due to impaired sexual functioning |

### IV. Perform/Provide:
| | |
|---|---|
| A. Opportunity for expression of fears regarding sexuality | A. Fosters open communication |

### V. Teach patient/family:
| | |
|---|---|
| A. Importance of communication with significant other | A. ↓ anxiety that may affect sexual functioning |

# ■ Cystitis

**DEFINITION:** The inflammation of the urinary bladder caused by the introduction of bacteria by way of a catheter, instrument, or by urinary retention

**CONCEPT/NEED:** Pain

**NURSING DIAGNOSIS:** Alteration in comfort: pain related to pressure of urination

**GOAL:** Increased comfort as evidenced by: verbalization, pulse WNL, ability to sleep all night

| INTERVENTION | RATIONALE |
|---|---|
| **II. Assess for:** | |
| A. Renal system assessment to include history and physical examination | A. Needed for data base |
| B. Pain, burning on urination, suprapubic and perineal pain due to spasm | B. Indicates infection |
| C. Frequency and urgency of urination and dribbling | C. Indicates infection |
| **III. Administer:** | |
| A. Analgesics as ordered | A. For control of pain |
| B. Antispasmodics as ordered | B. Relieves pain and urgency |
| **IV. Perform/Provide:** | |
| A. Heat to perineum | A. Reduces pain |
| B. Surgical removal of bladder obstruction is performed if needed (See Post-Operative Care, p. 17) | B. Cystitis may be caused by bladder calculus or neoplasm |
| **V. Teach patient/family:** | |
| A. Report recurrence of pain, frequency, and urgency | A. Prompt treatment of symptoms |

**CONCEPT/NEED:** Learning/Inflammation

**NURSING DIAGNOSIS:** Knowledge deficit of preventive measures related to denial

**GOAL:** Adequate knowledge of preventive measures as evidenced by: negative urine culture

| INTERVENTION | RATIONALE |
|---|---|
| **I. Monitor, describe, record:** | |
| A. I&O q 8 hr | A. Indicates fluid status |
| B. Temperature q 4 hr and PRN | B. Indicates infection |
| **II. Assess for:** | |
| A. Pyuria | A. Indicates infection |
| B. Hematuria | B. Indicates severe cystitis |
| C. Usual patterns of perineal care | C. May need teaching |
| D. Concentrated or cloudy urine | D. Beginning infection |
| E. Foul-smelling urine | E. May be present depending on organism |
| F. Urine culture and sensitivity | F. Reveals the causative organism and its antibiotic sensitivity |
| **III. Administer:** | |
| A. Urinary antiseptics as ordered | A. ↓ infection |
| B. Broad-spectrum antibiotics as ordered | B. ↓ infection |
| **IV. Perform/Provide:** | |
| A. Rest | A. During the acute phase |
| B. Increasing fluids | B. Promotes renal blood flow and flushes out bacteria |
| **V. Teach patient/family:** | |
| A. Basic knowledge about disease process and its causes | A. Helps prevent recurrence |
| B. Female patients wipe from front to back after urinating | B. ↓ infections from transfer of organisms |
| C. Empty bladder before and after intercourse | C. Washes ascending microbes away |

D. Avoid tub baths, shower with antibacterial soap

E. Avoid use of feminine hygiene sprays, strong soaps

F. Wear cotton underpants

G. Avoid prolonged bladder distention

H. Have follow-up urine studies

D. ↓ chance of infection

E. Interferes with normal flora

F. ↓ perineal moisture next to skin

G. Pooled urine good media for pathogens

H. Determines if asymptomatic infection is present

# ■ Glomerulonephritis/ Pyelonephritis

**DEFINITION:** Glomerulonephritis is a group of kidney diseases that involves an inflammatory or allergic reaction of the glomeruli usually caused by a streptoccocal infection. Usually confined to children and young adults. Pyelonephritis is the acute or chronic inflammation of the renal pelvis and tubules caused by bacterial infection usually as a result of cystitis or obstruction in the urinary tract

**CONCEPT/NEED:** Infection/Inflammation

**NURSING DIAGNOSIS:** Potential infection related to urinary retention

**GOAL:** Decreased infection as evidenced by: temperature WNL, absence of chills

| INTERVENTION | RATIONALE |
|---|---|
| **I. Monitor, describe, record:** | |
|   A. Temperature q 4 hr and PRN | A. Sign of infection |
| **II. Assess:** | |
|   A. Renal assessment to include history and physical exam | A. In pyleonephritis slightly rigid abdomen, kidney may be palpable |
|   B. History of recent streptococcal infections | B. Often a forerunner of this disorder |
|   C. Dull, bilateral loin pain | C. Symptom of this disorder |
|   D. Headache | D. Symptom of this disorder |
|   E. Low grade fever, chills | E. Symptoms of this disorder |
|   F. Urography, ureterography, cystography, and cystourethrography | F. Reveals obstruction location |
|   G. Antistreptolysin O titer | G. Increased in this disorder |
|   H. Microscopic examination of urine and urine culture | H. Casts in urine may reveal causative organism |
|   I. WBC | I. Increased leukocytes |

|                                          |                                                     |
| ---------------------------------------- | --------------------------------------------------- |
| J. Immunofluorescent staining            | J. Bacteria coated with immunoglobulin              |

### III. Administer:

|                                          |                                                     |
| ---------------------------------------- | --------------------------------------------------- |
| A. Antibiotics as ordered                | A. Eliminates infection and prevents re-infection   |
| B. Antipyretics as ordered               | B. ↓ fever                                           |
| C. Steroids as ordered                   | C. ↓ inflammation                                    |

### IV. Perform/Provide:

|                                          |                                                     |
| ---------------------------------------- | --------------------------------------------------- |
| A. Sterile technique for all procedures  | A. Patient is prone to infection                    |
| B. Restrict visitors with infections     | B. Prevents cross-infection                         |
| C. Bed bath with antibacterial soap      | C. Prevents infection                               |
| D. Bedrest with sedentary activities     | D. ↓ boredom, ↑ comfort during bedrest              |

### V. Teach patient/family:

|                                          |                                                     |
| ---------------------------------------- | --------------------------------------------------- |
| A. Avoid crowds, chilling, and persons with infections | A. If infection develops it may further injure the glomeruli |
| B. Report increased temperature, sore throat, flu, or cough | B. Symptoms of infection               |
| C. (See Teach patient/family in Cystitis under Inflammation/Infection, p. 279) | C. Urinary tract infections may further injure the glomeruli |

---

**CONCEPT/NEED:** Fluid/Electrolyte balance

**NURSING DIAGNOSIS:** Fluid volume excess related to decreased output

**GOAL:** Adequate fluid volume as evidenced by: no edema, electrolytes WNL

### INTERVENTION

### RATIONALE

### I. Monitor, describe, record:

|                                          |                                                     |
| ---------------------------------------- | --------------------------------------------------- |
| A. I&O q 8 hr                            | A. Evaluates fluid status                           |
| B. WT with same scale, clothing QID      | B. Insures adequate weight                          |

## II. Assess for:

A. Renal assessment to include history and physical assessment

A. Needed for data base

B. Scant smoky or bloody urine

B. Indicates renal shutdown

C. Oliguria and nocturia

C. Oliguria may result in potassium intoxication

D. Retinal edema, facial swelling, or swollen ankles

D. From fluid retention

E. Lethargy, arrhythmias, and impaired ventilation

E. S&S of hypokalemia

F. Muscle cramps, nausea, and colicky pain

F. S&S of hyperkalemia

G. Anemia

G. From azotemia

H. Anorexia, weight loss

H. From nausea, vomiting

I. Microscopic examination of urine

I. Renal epithelial cells

J. Specific gravity of urine

J. ↑ level

K. Sodium and potassium lab reports

K. May indicate electrolyte imbalance

## III. Administer:

A. Peritoneal dialysis or hemodialysis as ordered

A. ↓ impurities

B. Diuretics as ordered

B. Controls edema

C. Specific gravity of urine

C. ↑ level in this disorder

D. Needle biopsy assistance

D. Obstruction of glomerular capillaries

E. Parenteral fluid as ordered

E. May need controlled amounts

## IV. Perform/Provide:

A. Low sodium, high carbohydrate, low regular protein, low potassium diet as ordered

A. Carbohydrates increase energy and reduce protein catabolism in glomerulonephritis, regular protein diet in pyelonephritis

## V. Teach patient/family:

A. Reason for dietary and fluid restrictions

A. ↓ fluid retention

B. Report any sudden increase in weight

B. Sign of increased fluid retention

| | |
|---|---|
| C. Weigh daily at the same time with same scale | C. Observe any weight gain |
| D. Report puffy eyes and swollen extremities | D. Increased edema |
| E. Report decreased urinary output. Measure and record intake and output | E. May indicate renal shutdown. Needed to prevent complications |

---

**CONCEPT/NEED:** Transport/Circulation

**NURSING DIAGNOSIS:** Alteration in cardiac output related to fluid retention

**GOAL:** Decreased cardiac output as evidenced by: BP WNL

### INTERVENTION

### RATIONALE

**I. Monitor, describe, record:**
  A. BP q 4 hr and PRN

A. For hypertension

**II. Assess for:**
  A. Confusion, dizziness, or disorientation
  B. PPT and signs of CHF
  C. Renal failure and hypertensive encephalopathy

A. Related to hypertension or metabolic encephalopathy
B. If anticoagulant therapy is used
C. Low output with increased BP

**III. Administer:**
  A. Antihypertensive agents as ordered
  B. Anticoagulants as ordered

A. ↓ hypertension

B. Prevents thrombosis

**IV. Perform/Provide:**
  A. Restricted fluid intake
  B. Provide bedrest and restrict activities

A. ↓ hypertension
B. ↓ BP

**V. Teach patient/family:**
  A. How to take BP QID at the same time, position, and arm. Record BP accurately

A. Maintains correct record of BP

B. Report elevated BP

C. Name of all medications, purpose, side effects, and dosage

D. Need to avoid OTC medications

E. Rise to standing position slowly

B. Changes in therapeutic treatment may be required

C. Helps insure safe administration

D. May interact negatively with medications

E. Avoids hypotension and dizziness

# ■ Intravenous Therapy

**DEFINITION:** The administration of fluids, electrolytes, medications, and/or nutrients through a vein for rapid replacement and increase in blood volume

## INTERVENTION

### I. Monitor, describe, record:
A. Drip rate according to calculations and site q 30 min
B. Infiltration of fluids or medications causing swelling, pain, hematoma, redness
C. Thrombophlebitis from trauma to the vein
D. Symptoms of fluid overinfusion or underinfusion such as WT gain, edema, dyspnea, cough, sweating or WT loss, thirst, weakness, poor skin turgor, and oliguria
E. Symptoms of pyrogenic reaction such as temperature, headache, nausea, vomiting
F. Cannula and administration set replacement according to policy
G. Bags or flasks for leaks, cloudy solutions
H. I&O q 8 hr
I. VS q 4 hr

### II. Assess for:
A. Choice of site in arm or hand depending on time requirement of therapy
B. Previous reactions to IV therapy
C. Patient's knowledge of the procedure
D. Type of cannula to be used and size
E. Type of solution and tubing set-up to use
F. Additive solutions as ordered
G. Patient's parenteral fluid requirements
H. Patient's nutritional requirements

### III. Perform/Provide:
A. Venipuncture carrying out aseptic technique
B. Calculation of drip rate/min and time
C. Comfortable position for patient

D. Arm board or restraint if needed
E. Information to patient of steps in procedure and reason for therapy and to report pain or swelling
F. Safe removal of cannula when IV completed
G. Daily WT at same time, scale, and clothing

# ■ Nephrectomy/Nephrostomy

**DEFINITION:** Nephrostomy is the surgical incision into the kidney for removal of calculi or insertion of a tube for drainage. Nephrectomy is the surgical removal of a kidney as a result of tumor, injury or chronic conditions rendering the kidney nonfunctional or donation

**CONCEPT/NEED:** Learning

**NURSING DIAGNOSIS:** Knowledge deficit related to operative phase

**GOAL:** Increased knowledge as evidenced by: answering questions regarding surgery, stating he/she feels prepared for surgery

| INTERVENTION | RATIONALE |
|---|---|
| **II. Assess for:** | |
| A. Amount of knowledge regarding surgery, kidneys and their disease process, and expectations regarding outcome | A. Needed before beginning to teach |
| B. Amount of knowledge regarding possible infection (See Post-Operative Care, p. 17) | B. Insures safety |
| **V. Teach patient/family:** | |
| A. Renal function can be maintained by a single healthy kidney | A. ↓ anxiety |
| B. Avoid persons with URI or infections | B. Helps prevent infections |
| C. (See Pre-Operative Care, p. 13) | C. Assures that teaching to prevent post-op complications is done |

**CONCEPT/NEED:** Anxiety

**NURSING DIAGNOSIS:** Anxiety related to possible death

**GOAL:** Decreased anxiety as evidenced by: verbalization, ability to sleep at night, pulse WNL

| INTERVENTION | RATIONALE |
|---|---|
| **II. Assess for:** | |
| A. Verbal and nonverbal clues to anxiety | A. Patient may be unable to express feelings openly |
| B. Depression, grief, sadness | B. Mourning for lost kidney and altered body image |
| C. Pressure by family or guilt to donate a kidney | C. May influence self-image |
| D. Fear of illness, death, or decreased sexuality by donor | D. Common feelings of donors |
| E. Personal resources to cope with stress, e.g., significant other, financial status, previous surgical experience (See Psychosocial Assessment, p. 32) | E. Provides emotional support |
| **III. Administer:** | |
| A. Sedatives and tranquilizers as ordered | A. ↓ mental and emotional tension |
| **IV. Perform/Provide:** | |
| A. Comfortable quiet environment | A. ↓ anxiety |
| B. Explanations about equipment, lab tests, and personnel | B. Reassurance reduces anxiety |
| C. Opportunity for expression of fear of surgery, grieving for lost body part, and for questions | C. Fosters open communication |
| D. Stay with patient during periods of emotional crisis | D. Provides emotional support |
| E. Encourage participation in self-care as allowed by activity restrictions | E. Lessens sense of helplessness |
| **V. Teach patient/family:** | |
| A. Importance of communication with significant others | A. Provides for a release of tension and anxiety |

| | |
|---|---|
| B. Expect grief and mourning over loss of kidney | B. Important for good mental health |

---

**CONCEPT/NEED:** Pain

**NURSING DIAGNOSIS:** Alteration in comfort: pain related to incision

**GOAL:** Increased comfort as evidenced by: verbalization, decreasing request for pain medication, no grimacing

| INTERVENTION | RATIONALE |
|---|---|
| **II. Assess for:** | |
| A. Pain at site of incision | A. Needed for data base |
| B. Effectiveness of pain relief measures | B. May need more or less pain relief |
| C. Colicky-type pain (See Post-Operative Care, p. 17) | C. Due to passage of clots/obstruction |
| **III. Administer:** | |
| A. Narcotics or analgesics as ordered | A. Controls pain |
| **IV. Perform/Provide:** | |
| A. Position patient on back or operative side whenever possible | A. ↑ comfort |
| B. Offer medications for pain before ambulation | B. Minimizes pain |
| **V. Teach patient/family:** | |
| A. Report increased pain | A. May indicate complication |

---

**CONCEPT/NEED:** Fluid balance

**NURSING DIAGNOSIS:** Fluid volume excess related to decreased urinary output

**GOAL:** Adequate fluid volume as evidenced by: urine output 40–50 cc/hr, absence of edema

| INTERVENTION | RATIONALE |
|---|---|
| **I. Monitor, describe, record:** | |
| A. I&O q 8 hr as needed | A. Report output of 200 ml/8 hr or less |
| B. WT, QD same scale, time, clothes | B. Determines fluid retention |
| **II. Assess for:** | |
| A. Character and amount of urine | A. Pyuria, oliguria are signs of complications |
| B. Skin turgor | B. Determines status of fluid balance |
| C. Serum electrolyte studies, BUN, serum creatinine, intravenous urogram, radioisotope renography preoperatively | C. Assesses functional status and location of urinary tract and kidney |
| **III. Administer:** | |
| A. Parenteral fluids as ordered | A. Maintains fluid status |
| **IV. Perform/Provide:** | |
| A. Tape indwelling catheter to thigh | A. Relieves traction on bladder |
| B. FF to 3000 ml daily unless contraindicated | B. Insures proper fluids |
| C. FF prior to surgery, 1500–2000 cc from 8:00–12:00 PM night before surgery unless contraindicated | C. In donor nephrectomy |
| **V. Teach patient/family:** | |
| A. FF to 3000 ml daily | A. Needed for proper fluids |
| B. Report any increase/decrease in urine output | B. Insures safety |

# ■ Renal Calculi/Urolithiasis

**DEFINITION:** Stones in the renal system formed by crystalline substances excreted in the urine usually as a result of infection, immobility, urinary stasis, hypercalcemia, and hypercalciuria

**CONCEPT/NEED:** Pain

**NURSING DIAGNOSIS:** Alteration in comfort: pain related to obstruction

**GOAL:** Increased comfort as evidenced by: verbalization, requesting less pain medication, no grimacing

| INTERVENTION | RATIONALE |
|---|---|
| **II. Assess for:** | |
| A. Renal assessment to include history and physical examination | A. Needed for data base |
| B. Dull pain in loin or back | B. Stones in the calyces or renal pelvis |
| C. Excruciating flank pain radiating into the groin and testes or labia | C. Ureteral stones |
| D. Associated symptoms of pain, pallor, syncope, shock, nausea, and vomiting | D. Ureteral stones |
| E. Urinalysis | E. Presence of erythrocytes indicates injury by stones |
| F. Intravenous pyelography | F. Location of nonopaque stones, site and degree of obstruction |
| G. X-ray examination (KUB) | G. Presence of radiopaque stones |
| H. Physical and chemical analysis of calculus | H. Reveals composition of stones |
| I. Abrupt cessation of pain | I. Passage of stone |
| J. Increased flank pain | J. Sign of urinary obstruction |
| **III. Administer:** | |
| A. Narcotics as ordered | A. For control of pain |

## IV. Perform/Provide:

| | |
|---|---|
| A. Stay with patient during periods of severe pain | A. Provides emotional support |
| B. Warm soaks to affected flank | B. ↓ spasm |
| C. Filter all urine though gauze, inspect clots for presence of stone | C. Retain for analysis |
| D. Encourage ambulation with assistance (See Post-Operative Care, p. 17) | D. Promotes passage of stone |

## V. Teach patient/family:

| | |
|---|---|
| A. Importance of saving all urine | A. Passage of stone is not missed |

---

**CONCEPT/NEED:** Infection/Inflammation

**NURSING DIAGNOSIS:** Potential infection related to obstruction

**GOAL:** Absence of infection as evidenced by: temperature WNL, absence of chills, urine culture—negative

## INTERVENTION          RATIONALE

### I. Monitor, describe, record:

| | |
|---|---|
| A. Temperature q 4 hr and PRN | A. May indicate infection |

### II. Assess for:

| | |
|---|---|
| A. Elevated temperature, chills, dysuria, pyuria, frequency and urgency of urination | A. S&S of UTI |
| B. Urinalysis | B. Leukocytes present in infection |
| C. Urine culture | C. Causative organism |
| D. Urine for color and odor | D. Foul odor may accompany infection |

### III. Administer:

| | |
|---|---|
| A. Antibiotics as ordered | A. Treatment of infection |

## IV. Perform/Provide:

A. Strict aseptic technique in catheter care

A. Organisms may ascend tubing in UTI

## V. Teach patient/family:

A. Observe urine
(See Teach Patient/Family in Cystitis under Inflammation/Infection, p. 279)

A. For pus or odor

---

**CONCEPT/NEED:** Fluid balance

**NURSING DIAGNOSIS:** Fluid volume deficit related to abnormal fluid loss

**GOAL:** Adequate fluid balance as evidenced by: absence of edema, fluid intake of 3000 cc/day, good skin turgor

## INTERVENTION

## RATIONALE

### II. Assess for:

A. Usual fluid patterns
B. Nausea and vomiting
C. Physical and chemical analysis of calculus
D. Urinalysis, specific gravity

A. Needed for data base
B. Loss of fluids
C. Reveals composition of stones

D. Abnormal pH, either acidic or alkaline, increased specific gravity, high levels of uric acid, cystine, oxalate, calcium, phosphorus

E. Blood chemistry

E. Abnormal level of calcium, phosphorus, phosphatase, creatinine indicate reduced renal function

### IV. Perform/Provide:

A. Adequate fluids 2000–3000 ml/day
B. Parenteral fluids as ordered

A. Dilutes urine and prevents dehydration
B. ↑ hydrostatic pressure behind stone

## V. Teach patient/family:

A. Maintain fluid intake

A. Dilutes urine and prevents dehydration

B. Avoid all milk, chocolate, and nut products

B. Prevents calcium or phosphorous stones

C. Drink cranberry juice during infection

C. Forms an acid urine

D. Acid-ash diet

D. Forms slightly acid urine to prevent phosphate stone

# ■ Urinary Catheter

**DEFINITION:** Insertion of a tube to drain urine from the bladder when there is an obstruction, an inability to void, for incontinency, or following surgery on the bladder, prostate, or vagina. May be a single catheterization, an indwelling catheter, or a suprapubic catheter

## INTERVENTION

### I. Monitor, record:
  A. I&O q 8 hr
  B. Symptoms of infection such as cloudy urine, temperature elevation, chills, malaise
  C. Patency of tubing and correct attachment of catheter to leg to prevent backflow or traction on the urethra
  D. Results of urine cultures and urinalysis
  E. Drainage bag below level of bladder, no twisting or kinking of tubing, bag not to touch floor and emptied before too full
  F. Cleanliness and care of meatal area BID
  G. Complaints of pain
  H. VS q 4 hr

### II. Assess for:
  A. Size and type of catheter needed
  B. Voiding pattern, history of urinary tract problems
  C. Patient's knowledge of the procedure and why being done
  D. Distended bladder
  E. Dampness of skin or bed from incontinence

### III. Administer:
  A. Bacteriostatic ointment to meatus according to policy

### IV. Perform/Provide:
  A. Catheterization using aseptic technique and considering privacy
  B. Connection to closed drainage system or irrigation system
  C. Change of catheter according to policy
  D. Information to patient of steps in procedure and reason for procedure
  E. Safe removal of catheter when disconnected
  F. Increased fluid intake to 3000 ml/day

### V. Teach patient/family:
  A. Importance of activity, personal cleanliness

B. Clean area around catheter
C. Empty bag q 2 hr
D. Connect catheter to bag
E. Maintain patency of tubing
F. Prevent urine backflow
G. Increase daily fluid intake
H. Report to physician if catheter comes out, pain, no urine, cloudy urine, elevated temperature
I. Self-administration of medicines and check before taking OTC drugs

# MUSCULOSKELETAL SYSTEM STANDARDS

- Musculoskeletal System Assessment
- Amputation/Upper and Lower Extremity
- Cast/Traction
- Fractures
- Gout
- Laminectomy/Lumbar, Cervical, Spinal Fusion
- Low Back Pain
- Lupus Erythematosus
- Osteoarthritis/Degenerative Joint Disease
- Osteomyelitis
- Osteoporosis
- Rheumatoid Arthritis
- Total Hip or Knee Replacement/Hip or Knee Arthroplasty

# ■ Musculoskeletal System Assessment

**DEFINITION:** The collection of data concerning the musculoskeletal system and its functional capabilities to be used in identifying nursing problems related to mobility and activity

## INTERVENTION

I. **Interview and investigate for and record past history:**
   A. Previous bone, joint, or muscle conditions such as arthritis, bursitis, fractures, gout, low back pain, ruptured disk, nerve impairment, muscle deterioration, poliomyelitis
   B. Family members with joint or bone diseases
   C. Previous operations, injuries, or other medical conditions related to bones, joints such as spinal or orthopedic surgery, muscular dystrophy, multiple sclerosis, cerebral palsy
   D. Alcohol, smoking, chemical ingestion
   E. Exposure to hazardous condition, proneness to accidents
   F. Poor coordination in walking or other movements, pain or swelling, in joints, changes in ROM and activity, cramps, weakness or twitching of muscles, ability to sit, stand, walk, grasp, climb stairs walk, grasp, climb stairs
   G. Usual amount of activity, kind and frequency per day
   H. Customary medications taken for pain or other, and response
   I. Past blood, urine x-ray tests of bones, scans, aspiration of joint, myelogram, CAT or other tests, and results

II. **Interview and investigate for and record present history:**
   A. Chief complaint
   B. Onset and length of illness
   C. Knowledge of disease, procedures, and planned therapy
   D. Use of trapeze, cast, traction application
   E. Results of urinalysis, CBC, calcium, phosphorus, scans, myelograms, x-ray, aspirations, biopsy done
   F. Medications taken for a musculoskeletal problem
   G. Bedrest, chair, bathroom privileges, or amount of activity allowed

III. **Inspection for:**
   A. ROM of all joints, degree of motion

B. Ability to sit, lie, get up, stand, walk, bend and posture, use hands and fingers, grasp, pinch, complete daily functions
C. Symmetry of extremities, shoulders, clavicles, scapulae, musculature
D. Deformities such as contractures, deviations, changes in contour, scoliosis, kyphosis, lordosis, claw or hammer toe, toeing in or toeing out
E. Joint or muscle pain, redness, swelling
F. Gait, coordination, supportive aids to ambulate, balance, endurance
G. Body alignment on supine, prone, side lying
H. Paralysis, amputation, casts, brace, traction

## IV. Palpation for:
A. Warmth at joints
B. Crepitus from joint motion
C. Muscle strength, mass, tone
D. Reflexes to include biceps, triceps, pectoralis, brachioradial, patellar, plantar
E. Tenderness upon pressure or movement
F. Thickening, bony enlargement around joints

# ■ Amputation/Upper and Lower Extremity

**DEFINITION:** The surgical removal of the total or part of the lower or upper extremity as a result of trauma, disease, or congenital deformity

**CONCEPT/NEED:** Anxiety

**NURSING DIAGNOSIS:** Anxiety related to loss of limb

**GOAL:** Reduced anxiety as evidenced by: verbalization, pulse WNL, ability to sleep at night

## INTERVENTION

II. **Assess for:**
   A. Verbal/nonverbal clues of anxiety
   B. Personal resources
   C. Response to information/ treatment
   D. Change in life-style
   E. Poor body image
   F. Knowledge of procedure

IV. **Perform/Provide:**
   A. Accepting environment
   B. Reduced anxiety-producing situations
   C. Referral for counseling if needed
   D. Assist in self-care if needed

V. **Teach patient/family:**
   A. Avoidance of anxiety-producing situations
   B. Possible changes in life-style

## RATIONALE

A. May be unable to openly communicate
B. Provides support
C. ↓ anxiety

D. May need to provide support
E. Due to loss
F. ↓ anxiety

A. Emotional support
B. ↓ anxiety

C. May need psychiatric intervention

D. ↑ self-confidence

A. ↓ anxiety

B. May need emotional support

**CONCEPT/NEED:** Learning

**NURSING DIAGNOSIS:** Knowledge deficit related to post-operative complications

**GOAL:** Adequate knowledge as evidenced by: stating he/she is willing to comply with instructions, ability to demonstrate pre-operative teaching

| INTERVENTION | RATIONALE |
|---|---|
| **II. Assess for:** | |
| A. Knowledge of post-op condition | A. ↓ recovery time, ↓ anxiety |
| B. Level of pre-op teaching | B. Needed for appropriate level of teaching |
| C. Physical preparation | C. Fluid and nutritional status must be optimum |
| **IV. Perform/Provide:** | |
| A. Clear, concise instructions for muscle exercise and crutch walking | A. For adequate understanding |
| B. Furniture moved to allow for crutches (See Post-Operative Care, p. 17) | B. Insures safety |
| **V. Teach patient/family:** | |
| A. About adherence to rehabilitation | A. ↓ recovery time |
| B. (See Pre-Operative Care, p. 13) | B. Perform pre-operative teaching |

---

**CONCEPT/NEED:** Pain

**NURSING DIAGNOSIS:** Alteration in comfort: pain related to incision

**GOAL:** Pain reduced as evidenced by: verbalization, decreased request for pain medication

| INTERVENTION | RATIONALE |
|---|---|
| **II. Assess for:** | |
| A. Characteristics of pain, type, location | A. Needed for data base |
| B. Any associated symptoms of pain | B. Excessive anxiety may increase pain |
| C. Conditions which relieve pain | C. Needed for data base |
| D. Precipitating factors of pain | D. May need to decrease these |
| **III. Administer:** | |
| A. Analgesics as ordered | A. ↓ pain |
| **IV. Perform/Provide:** | |
| A. Positioning q 2 hr | A. ↑ comfort |
| B. Turning BID X 30 min, prone for lower extremities (See Cast Care for turning, p. 307) | B. Prevents flexion contractures |
| **V. Teach patient/family:** | |
| A. Importance of proper body alignment | A. Promotes comfort |
| B. Phantom pain can be expected | B. ↓ anxiety over pain |

---

**CONCEPT/NEED:** Activity/Mobility

**NURSING DIAGNOSIS:** Activity intolerance related to pain

**GOAL:** Increasing mobility as evidenced by: progressive activity program

| INTERVENTION | RATIONALE |
|---|---|
| **I. Monitor, describe, record:** | |
| A. Daily pattern of activity | A. Needed for data base |

## II. Assess for:
| | |
|---|---|
| A. Skin breakdown | A. Result of immobility |

## III. Administer:
| | |
|---|---|
| A. Pain medications 1 hr before activity | A. ↑ comfort |

## IV. Perform/Provide:
| | |
|---|---|
| A. Active/passive ROM (See Cast/Traction Care, p. 307) | A. Prevents contractures |

## V. Teach patient/family:
| | |
|---|---|
| A. Importance of exercise/nutrition | A. Promotes healing |

---

**CONCEPT/NEED:** Grieving

**NURSING DIAGNOSIS:** Grieving related to loss of limb

**GOAL:** Adequate grieving as evidenced by: performing self-care, moving through the stages of denial, anger, depression, acceptance

### INTERVENTION

### RATIONALE

## II. Assess for:
| | |
|---|---|
| A. Excessive dependency | A. ↓ self-image |
| B. Adaptation to amputation | B. Needed for data base |
| C. Knowledge of community resources/support groups | C. Aids rehabilitation |

## IV. Perform/Provide:
| | |
|---|---|
| A. Encouragement in self-care | A. ↓ dependency |
| B. Information on support groups | B. Emotional support |

## V. Teach patient/family:
| | |
|---|---|
| A. Family to provide listening atmosphere | A. Emotional support |
| B. Necessity of exercises/follow-up care | B. Insures adherence |

# ■ Cast/Traction

**DEFINITION:** A cast is a device made of plaster material applied to a part of the body for purposes of immobilization, protection, and support during healing and the prevention or correction of a deformity. Traction is a method of providing a pulling force in two directions to a part of the body for the purpose of immobilization, reduction, and alignment and to prevent deformity

## INTERVENTION

### I. Monitor, describe, record:
  A. VS q 4 hr and PRN
  B. Pulses in extremity affected, q 4 hr and PRN
  C. Proper weights on traction
  D. Neurovascular status q 4–24 hr and PRN
  E. Maintenance of ropes and pulleys
  F. Fluid/nutritional intake to include high protein, low carbohydrates, and upper limit of calculated fluid need

### II. Assess for:
  A. Impaired blood flow, nailbed refill, pallor or cyanosis of skin, coldness, swelling, numbness, toe or finger movement of affected part
  B. Pain in affected part and what relieves it
  C. Odor, drainage or bleeding, pressure or burning in affected part, pin site
  D. Loss of sensation, foot drop, paralysis
  E. Pressure on skin or bony parts, rubbing or irritation by cast, rashes, or itching
  F. Dryness, smoothness, tightness of cast
  G. Changes in elimination, rest pattern
  H. Amount and ability of movement in bed and self-care
  I. Alignment, support, bandages

### III. Administer:
  A. Analgesics for pain as ordered
  B. Stool softener or laxative as ordered
  C. Antibiotics as ordered

### IV. Perform/Provide:
  A. Daily skin care per assessment

B. Pin care BID
C. Active/passive exercises
D. Positioning q 2 hr
E. Bedrest with extremity elevated and/or proper amount of traction
F. Petal cast rough edges
G. Clean cast PRN
H. Bivalve cast if needed
I. Maintenance of weights and pulleys
J. Antiembolic hose, cough, deep breathe q 2–4 hr
K. Maintain alignment, ordered position
L. Diversional activities to decrease boredom
M. Ice application as ordered
N. Assistance with daily functions, ambulation
O. Clean, dry, wrinkle- and crumb-free linens

## V. Teach patient/family:
A. Value of exercises, movement, positioning
B. Crutch walking
C. Cast care and reporting of odors, drainage, pain, numbness, tingling, temperature
D. Skin care, clean, dry, lotions
E. Dietary and fluid intake

# ■ Fractures

**DEFINITION:** A break in a bone usually accompanied by surrounding soft tissue injury caused by an injury or disease process. May be complete, open, or closed

**CONCEPT/NEED:** Pain

**NURSING DIAGNOSIS:** Alteration in comfort: pain related to trauma

**GOAL:** Increased comfort as evidenced by: verbalization, decreasing request for pain medication

| INTERVENTION | RATIONALE |
|---|---|
| **II. Assess for:** | |
| A. Characteristics of pain, type, location | A. Needed for data base |
| B. Any associated symptoms of pain | B. Excessive anxiety may increase pain |
| C. Conditions which relieve pain | C. Needed for data base |
| D. Precipitating factors of pain | D. May need to decrease these |
| E. Proper support and alignment | E. Prevents complications |
| **III. Administer:** | |
| A. Analgesics, muscle relaxants as ordered | A. ↓ pain |
| B. Cold applications as ordered | B. ↓ inflammation |
| **IV. Perform/Provide:** | |
| A. Immobilization and elevation of limb | A. Prevents complications |
| B. Body alignment (See Cast/Traction Care, p. 307) | B. Promotes comfort |

## V. Teach patient/family:
A. Importance of proper body alignment    A. Promotes comfort

---

**CONCEPT/NEED:** Infection

**NURSING DIAGNOSIS:** Potential infection related to skin breakdown

**GOAL:** Absence of infection as evidenced by: no redness, purulent drainage, temperature WNL

| **INTERVENTION** | **RATIONALE** |
|---|---|
| **I. Monitor, describe, record:** | |
| A. Temperature q 4 hr | A. Indicates infection |
| **II. Assess for:** | |
| A. Edema, heat of affected limbs | A. Indicates infection |
| B. WBC elevation | B. Indicates infection |
| **III. Administer:** | |
| A. Antibiotics as ordered | A. ↓ infection |

---

**CONCEPT/NEED:** Transport/Circulation

**NURSING DIAGNOSIS:** Alteration in cardiac output: decreased related to obstruction

**GOAL:** Adequate cardiac output as evidenced by: RBC, Hct WNL, BP WNL

| **INTERVENTION** | **RATIONALE** |
|---|---|
| **I. Monitor, describe, record:** | |
| A. VS q 15 min | A. Indicates circulation |
| B. Peripheral pulses distal to injury | B. Indicates circulation |

## II. Assess for:

| | |
|---|---|
| A. Changes in color, sensation, temperature | A. Indicates circulation |
| B. Tingling, numbness, burning, pain | B. Possible nerve damage |
| C. Coldness, cyanosis, swelling below cast | C. Possible ischemic paralysis |
| D. Extent, type of blood loss | D. Possible hemorrhage |
| E. Chest pain, pallor, dyspnea, petechial hemorrhage | E. Possible fat embolism |

## III. Administer:

| | |
|---|---|
| A. Blood components/volume expanders | A. ↑ blood volume |
| B. O₂ as ordered | B. ↓ local anoxia |
| C. IV fluids as ordered | C. Emulsifying effect |
| D. Casts, splints, traction as needed | D. For immobilization |

## IV. Perform/Provide:

| | |
|---|---|
| A. High Fowler's position | A. ↑ O₂, circulation |

## V. Teach patient/family:

| | |
|---|---|
| A. Report increased pain, loss of sensation in extremities | A. Possible complications |

---

**CONCEPT/NEED:** Activity

**NURSING DIAGNOSIS:** Activity intolerance related to pain

**GOAL:** Increased activity as evidenced by: progressive activity program

| **INTERVENTION** | **RATIONALE** |
|---|---|
| **II. Assess for:** | |
| A. ROM q 4 hr | A. Prevents contractures |
| **III. Administer:** | |
| A. Pain medication before activity | A. ↓ pain |

**IV. Perform/Provide:**
    A. Assist in daily functions    A. ↓ anxiety
    B. Quiet calm environment    B. ↓ anxiety

**V. Teach patient/family:**
    A. Importance of ROM    A. Maintains muscle function
    B. Relaxation exercises    B. ↓ anxiety

# ■ Gout

**DEFINITION:** A metabolic disorder resulting in deposits of uric acid crystals in joints and connective tissues causing pain, swelling, inflammation

**CONCEPT/NEED:** Pain

**NURSING DIAGNOSIS:** Alteration in comfort: pain related to inflammation

**GOAL:** Increased comfort as evidenced by: verbalization, reduced request for pain medications

## INTERVENTION

II. **Assess for:**
   A. Characteristics of pain, type, location
   B. Warm dusty red, purple skin around joint
   C. Inflammation of joints
   D. Pruritus/desquamation of area
   E. WBC, ESR, BUN, $Na^+$ urate crystals in joint fluids
   F. Family history of gout

III. **Administer:**
   A. Antigout agents as ordered
   B. Cold/heat applications as ordered
   C. Steroids as ordered

IV. **Perform/Provide:**
   A. Bedrest for acute attack
   B. Position of comfort
   C. Bed cradle
   D. ROM q 4 hr

## RATIONALE

A. Needed for data base

B. Indicates gout

C. Indicates gout
D. Indicates recovery from gout

E. Increased in gout

F. Hereditary

A. ↓ uric acid
B. ↓ inflammation

C. ↓ inflammation

A. ↓ edema
B. Promotes comfort
C. ↓ WT on area
D. ↓ venous stasis

## V. Teach patient/family:

A. Avoid aspirin products

A. Antagonist to antigout medications

B. Prescribed medications, names, dosage, times, purpose, side effects

B. Insures safety

---

**CONCEPT/NEED:** Nutrition

**NURSING DIAGNOSIS:** Alteration in nutrition: more than body requirements related to increased intake (purines)

**GOAL:** Adequate nutrition as evidenced by: eating a low purine diet

## INTERVENTION

## RATIONALE

### II. Assess for:
A. Diet low in purines

A. Uric acid is end product of purines

B. Calculi in urine
C. Alkalinity of urine
D. Usual nutritional pattern

B. Urate crystals may be in urine
C. Inhibits calculi
D. Needed for data base

### III. Administer:
A. Diet low in purines

A. ↓ uric acid

### IV. Perform/Provide:
A. Basic information about condition

A. ↓ anxiety

B. Adequate fluids
C. Test for pH of urine

B. ↓ renal calculi
C. Increased pH decreases renal calculi

### V. Teach patient/family:
A. Avoid foods high in purines
B. Procedure for pH of urine

A. ↓ uric acid
B. Insures accurate results

# ■ Laminectomy/Lumbar, Cervical, Spinal Fusion

**DEFINITION:** A surgical procedure on the lumbar or cervical vertebrae done to relieve pressure on the spinal nerves resulting from herniated disk, trauma, or disease

**CONCEPT/NEED:** Anxiety

**NURSING DIAGNOSIS:** Anxiety related to surgery

**GOAL:** Reduced anxiety as evidenced by: verbalization, pulse WNL

| INTERVENTION | RATIONALE |
|---|---|
| **II. Assess for:** | |
| A. Verbal/nonverbal clues to anxiety | A. May not be able to express feelings openly |
| B. Knowledge level of disease process | B. Needed for data base |
| **III. Administer:** | |
| A. Anti-anxiety drugs as ordered | A. ↓ anxiety |
| **IV. Perform/Provide:** | |
| A. Emotional support | A. ↓ anxiety |
| B. Quiet calm environment | B. ↓ anxiety |
| **V. Teach patient/family:** | |
| A. About surgery (See Pre-Operative Care, p. 13) | A. ↓ anxiety |
| B. Relaxation exercises | B. ↓ anxiety |

**CONCEPT/NEED:** Pain

**NURSING DIAGNOSIS:** Alteration in comfort: pain related to inflammation

**GOAL:** Increased comfort as evidenced by: verbalization, reduced request for pain medication

| INTERVENTION | RATIONALE |
|---|---|
| II. **Assess for:** | |
| A. Characteristics of pain, type, location | A. Needed for data base |
| B. Sensation of extremities post-op | B. Post-op neurological complication |
| III. **Administer:** | |
| A. Analgesics as ordered | A. ↓ pain |
| IV. **Perform/Provide:** | |
| A. Proper body alignment | A. Promotes comfort |
| B. Log rolling when turning | B. Prevents twisting back |
| V. **Teach patient/family:** | |
| A. Proper body alignment | A. Pain control |

---

**CONCEPT/NEED:** Transport/Circulation

**NURSING DIAGNOSIS:** Alteration in cardiac output related to blood loss

**GOAL:** Adequate cardiac output as evidenced by: BP WNL, absence of frank blood

| INTERVENTION | RATIONALE |
|---|---|
| I. **Monitor, describe, record:** | |
| A. VS q 4 hr | A. May indicate complication |
| B. Color, temperature and sensation in extremity | B. Indicates circulation |
| II. **Assess for:** | |
| A. Blood loss | A. Possible hemorrhage |
| III. **Administer:** | |
| A. Fluids as ordered | A. Replenishes blood loss |

## IV. Perform/Provide:

A. Circulation checks q 4 hr (See Cast/Traction Care, p. 307)

A. Cast may interfere with circulation

B. Active/passive ROM

B. ↑ circulation

# ■ Low Back Pain

**DEFINITION:** Pain in the lumbar region of the back usually caused by musculoskeletal conditions such as a herniated disk degeneration

**CONCEPT/NEED:** Pain

**NURSING DIAGNOSIS:** Alteration in comfort: pain related to inflammation

**GOAL:** Increased comfort as evidenced by: verbalization, ability to sleep at night

| INTERVENTION | RATIONALE |
|---|---|
| **II. Assess for:** | |
| A. Characteristics of pain, type, location | A. Needed for data base |
| B. Any associated symptoms of pain | B. Excessive anxiety may increase pain |
| C. Conditions which relieve pain | C. Needed for data base |
| D. Precipitating factors of pain | D. May need to decrease these |
| E. Proper support and alignment | E. Prevents complications |
| F. Work history (See Work Assessment, p. 37) | F. May contribute to pain |
| **III. Administer:** | |
| A. Analgesics, muscle relaxants as ordered | A. ↓ pain |
| B. Cold/heat application as ordered | B. ↓ inflammation |
| **IV. Perform/Provide:** | |
| A. Body alignment | A. Promotes comfort |
| B. Pelvic traction as ordered | B. Relieves pressure on spinal nerve |

## V. Teach patient/family:

A. Importance of proper body alignment

A. Promotes comfort

B. Proper exercise program

B. Strengthens back

C. About medications, side effects, dosage, time

C. Insures safety

# ■ Lupus Erythematosus

**DEFINITION:** A systemic inflammatory autoimmune disease affecting the major systems and body organs

**CONCEPT/NEED:** Skin integrity

**NURSING DIAGNOSIS:** Impairment of skin integrity related to facial rash/lesions

**GOAL:** Skin integrity as evidenced by: absence of scales

| INTERVENTION | RATIONALE |
|---|---|
| **II. Assess for:** | |
| A. Butterfly rash on face or lesions on other areas | A. Present in half of cases |
| B. Verbal/nonverbal clues to lowered self-image | B. May be unable to communicate feelings |
| C. Level of knowledge of condition | C. Needed for teaching |
| **III. Administer:** | |
| A. Cool baths as ordered | A. Soothes the skin |
| B. Topical steroids | B. ↓ inflammation |
| C. Sunscreens | C. Sunlight aggravates condition |
| **IV. Perform/Provide:** | |
| A. Mouth care q 4 hr | A. For mouth lesions |
| B. Emotional support | B. ↑ self-image |
| **V. Teach patient/family:** | |
| A. Proper oral hygiene | A. ↓ bleeding gums |
| B. Cleaning of lesions with mild soap | B. Prevents infection |
| C. All aspects of condition | C. Insures safety |
| D. Avoidance of ultraviolet light, hair sprays | D. ↑ condition |
| E. Available lupus organizations | E. For emotional support |

**CONCEPT/NEED:** Pain

**NURSING DIAGNOSIS:** Alteration in comfort: pain related to inflammation

**GOAL:** Increased comfort as evidenced by: verbalization, reduced request for pain medication

| INTERVENTION | RATIONALE |
|---|---|
| **II. Assess for:** | |
| A. Characteristics of pain | A. Needed for data base |
| B. Swelling, redness, warmth of joints | B. Inflammatory reaction |
| C. Weakness, fatigue | C. Inflammatory reaction |
| D. Daily functions | D. May need to assist |
| **III. Administer:** | |
| A. Analgesics as ordered | A. For pain relief |
| B. Plasmapheresis as ordered | B. Immune complexes removed from blood |
| **IV. Perform/Provide:** | |
| A. Adequate rest | A. Prevents fatigue |
| B. Assistance for daily functions | B. Fatigue and immobility |
| **V. Teach patient/family:** | |
| A. About all medications, side effects, dosage, time | A. Insures safety |
| B. Importance of avoiding stress | B. Prevents episodes |

# ■ Osteoarthritis/Degenerative Joint Disease

**DEFINITION:** A chronic, localized, progressive disease of the joints (hip, feet, hands) resulting in erosion of the cartilage causing pain, muscle spasms, and limitations in physical activity

**CONCEPT/NEED:** Pain

**NURSING DIAGNOSIS:** Alteration in comfort: pain related to inflammation

**GOAL:** Increased comfort as evidenced by: verbalization, absence of grimacing

| INTERVENTION | RATIONALE |
|---|---|
| **II. Assess for:** | |
| A. Characteristics of pain, type, location | A. Needed for data base |
| B. Any associated symptoms of pain | B. Excessive anxiety may increase pain |
| C. Conditions which relieve pain | C. Needed for data base |
| D. Precipitating factors of pain | D. May need to decrease these |
| E. Proper support and alignment | E. Prevents complications |
| F. Work history (See Work Assessment, p. 37) | F. May contribute to pain |
| **III. Administer:** | |
| A. Analgesics, muscle relaxants as ordered | A. ↓ pain |
| B. Heat applications as ordered | B. ↓ inflammation |
| **IV. Perform/Provide:** | |
| A. Bedrest | A. Relieves pain |

B. Body alignment
C. ROM as tolerated

B. Promotes comfort
C. Prevents complications

## V. Teach patient/family:
A. Importance of proper body alignment

A. Promotes comfort

B. Proper exercise program

B. Strengthens joints

C. About medications, side effects, dosage, time

C. Insures safety

# ■ Osteomyelitis

**DEFINITION:** An infection of the bone caused by pathogenic organisms

**CONCEPT/NEED:** Pain

**NURSING DIAGNOSIS:** Alteration in comfort: pain related to inflammation

**GOAL:** Increased comfort as evidenced by: verbalization, reduced request for pain medication

| INTERVENTION | RATIONALE |
|---|---|
| **II. Assess for:** | |
| A. Characteristics of pain, type, location | A. Needed for data base |
| B. Any associated symptoms of pain | B. Excessive anxiety may increase pain |
| C. Conditions which relieve pain | C. Needed for data base |
| D. Precipitating factors of pain | D. May need to decrease these |
| E. Proper support and alignment | E. Prevents complications |
| **III. Administer:** | |
| A. Analgesics as ordered | A. ↓ pain |
| B. Heat applications as ordered | B. ↓ inflammation |
| **IV. Perform/Provide:** | |
| A. Bedrest | A. Relieves pain |
| B. Body alignment/elevation of limb | B. Promotes comfort |
| C. Dressing changes if indicated | C. Prevents infection |
| D. ROM BID | D. Prevents stiffness |

## V. Teach patient/family:

A. Importance of proper body alignment

B. Proper exercise program

C. About medications, side effects, dosage, time

A. Promotes comfort

B. Maintains mobility

C. Insures safety

# ■ Osteoporosis

**DEFINITION:** A bone metabolism disorder causing a decrease in bone mass and resulting in bone porosity and brittleness leading to fractures and deformities

**CONCEPT/NEED:** Safety

**NURSING DIAGNOSIS:** Potential for injury related to falls

**GOAL:** Absence of injury as evidenced by: absence of falls

## INTERVENTION

II. **Assess for:**
   A. Degree of immobility
   B. Daily pattern of activity

III. **Administer:**
   A. Calcitonin as ordered
   B. Diet high in calcium

IV. **Perform/Provide:**
   A. Active/passive ROM
   B. Back rubs and position change PRN

V. **Teach patient/family:**
   A. Importance of exercise/nutrition
   B. Prevention of falls

## RATIONALE

A. Needed for data base
B. Needed for data base

A. Prevents calcium loss
B. Insures calcium intake

A. Prevents contractures
B. Prevents skin breakdown

A. Prevents fractures/deformity

B. Prevents fractures

# ■ Rheumatoid Arthritis

**DEFINITION:** A chronic, systemic, progressive, and inflammatory disease affecting the synovial membrane of the joints causing pain, swelling, and deformities

**CONCEPT/NEED:** Pain

**NURSING DIAGNOSIS:** Alteration in comfort: pain related to inflammation

**GOAL:** Increased comfort as evidenced by: verbalization, absence of joint swelling, ability to move with ease

## INTERVENTION

II. **Assess for:**
   A. Characteristics of pain, type, location
   B. Any associated symptoms of pain
   C. Conditions which relieve pain
   D. Precipitating factors of pain
   E. Malaise, WT loss, paresthesis
   F. Subcutaneous nodules, weakness, fatigue, stiffness

III. **Administer:**
   A. Analgesics
   B. Heat/cold applications as ordered
   C. Gold compounds

IV. **Perform/Provide:**
   A. Bedrest
   B. Body alignment

## RATIONALE

A. Needed for data base

B. Excessive anxiety may increase pain
C. Needed for data base

D. May need to decrease these
E. Prodromal symptoms

F. Other symptoms

A. ↓ pain
B. ↓ inflammation

C. ↓ inflammation

A. Relieves pain
B. Promotes comfort

C. ROM as tolerated     C. Prevents complications
D. Bed cradle     D. Keeps linens off painful areas

## V. Teach patient/family:
A. Importance of proper body alignment     A. Promotes comfort
B. Proper exercise program     B. Strengthens joints
C. About medications, side effects, dosage, time     C. Insures safety
D. Avoid quick jerky movements     D. Pain avoidance

---

**CONCEPT/NEED:** Activity

**NURSING DIAGNOSIS:** Activity intolerance related to pain

**GOAL:** Adequate activity as evidenced by: no stiffness, contractures, normal daily functions

## INTERVENTION

## RATIONALE

### I. Monitor, describe, record:
A. VS q 4 hr     A. May indicate complication

### II. Assess for:
A. Degree of immobility     A. Needed for data base
B. Level of activity     B. Needed for data base
C. Daily pattern of activity     C. Needed for data base

### III. Administer:
A. Anti-arthritic medications     A. ↑ mobility

### IV. Perform/Provide:
A. Active/passive ROM     A. Prevents contractures
B. Back rubs and position change PRN     B. Prevents skin breakdown

### V. Teach patient/family:
A. Importance of exercise/nutrition     A. Promotes healing and mobility

# ■ Total Hip or Knee Replacement/ Hip or Knee Arthroplasty

**DEFINITION:** A surgical procedure that totally or partially replaces a hip or knee joint with an artificial joint and is performed to relieve pain and restore joint motion in selected patients with arthritis

**CONCEPT/NEED:** Pain

**NURSING DIAGNOSIS:** Alteration in comfort: pain related to incision

**GOAL:** Increased comfort as evidenced by: verbalization, absence of grimacing, ability to move without pain

| INTERVENTION | RATIONALE: |
|---|---|
| **II. Assess for:** | |
| A. Characteristics of pain, type, location | A. Needed for data base |
| B. Any associated symptoms of pain | B. Excessive anxiety may increase pain |
| C. Conditions which relieve pain | C. Needed for data base |
| D. Precipitating factors of pain | D. May need to decrease these |
| E. Edema, excessive fluids at site | E. Will cause pain |
| **III. Administer:** | |
| A. Analgesics | A. ↓ pain |
| B. Ice applications as ordered | B. ↓ inflammation |
| **IV. Perform/Provide:** | |
| A. Bedrest | A. Relieves pain |
| B. Body alignment | B. Promotes comfort |
| C. Suction of wound | C. Relieves pressure |

## V. Teach patient/family:
A. Importance of proper body A. Promotes comfort
   alignment

---

**CONCEPT/NEED:** Activity

**NURSING DIAGNOSIS:** Activity intolerance related to pain

**GOAL:** Adequate activity as evidenced by: progressive exercise program

## INTERVENTION

### RATIONALE

I. **Monitor, describe, record:**
   A. VS q 4 hr          A. May indicate complication

II. **Assess for:**
   A. Readiness to begin exercise   A. Needed for teaching
      program
   B. Level of activity         B. Needed for data base
   C. Daily pattern of activity    C. Needed for data base
   D. Skin breakdown       D. Result of immobility
   E. Proper positioning after   E. Held in abduction with splint,
      surgery             head of bed elevated less than 45
      (See Post-Operative Care, p.   degrees
      17)

IV. **Perform/Provide:**
   A. Active/passive ROM     A. Prevents contractures
   B. Back rubs and position   B. Prevents skin breakdown
      change PRN
   C. Position on unaffected side   C. Promotes healing

V. **Teach patient/family:**
   A. Importance of exercise    A. Promotes healing
   B. Remain with extremities ab-   B. Prevents dislocation of prosthesis
      ducted in hip flex less than
      45 degrees

---

**CONCEPT/NEED:** Infection

**NURSING DIAGNOSIS:** Potential infection related to contamination

**GOAL:** Infection will be prevented as evidenced by: Temperature WNL, no redness, purulent drainage

| INTERVENTION | RATIONALE |
|---|---|
| **II. Assess for:** | |
| A. VS q 4 hr | A. May indicate infection |
| B. Swelling, redness | B. Inflammatory reaction |
| C. Weakness, fatigue | C. Inflammatory reaction |
| **III. Administer:** | |
| A. Antibiotics as ordered | A. For infection |
| **IV. Perform/Provide:** | |
| A. Adequate rest | A. Prevents fatigue |
| B. Aseptic techniques, dressing changes | B. Prevents infection |
| **V. Teach patient/family:** | |
| A. About all medications, side effects, dosage, time | A. Insures safety |
| B. About signs of post-hospital infection | B. Prevents complications |

# REPRODUCTIVE SYSTEM STANDARDS

- Female Reproductive System Assessment
- Male Reproductive System Assessment
- Abdominal Hysterectomy/Bilateral Salpingo-Oophorectomy
- Abortion
- Dilation and Curettage/Conization of Cervix
- Radical Mastectomy/Simple Mastectomy
- Pelvic Inflammatory Disease
- Prostatectomy/Transurethral/Suprapubic/Retropubic
- Prostatic Hypertrophy/Prostatitis
- Tubal Ligation/Tubal Pregnancy
- Vaginal Hysterectomy/Anterior and Posterior Colporrhaphy

# ■ Female Reproductive System Assessment

**DEFINITION:** The collection of a data base concerning the female reproductive system and its functional capabilities to be used in identifying nursing problems related to sexuality, reproduction and elimination

## INTERVENTION

### I. Interview and investigate for and record past history:
A. Previous conditions such as venereal diseases, renal calculi, tubal pregnancy, PID, abortions, vaginal infections
B. Previous surgeries such as hysterectomy, D&C, mastectomy
C. Vaginal discharges, itching, pain or lesion of genitalia, rashes or irritations of genitalia
D. Difficulty in urination, starting, frequency or unable to empty bladder, incontinence or stress incontinence, burning or pain
E. Infertility problem, sexual difficulties, libido
F. Frequency of intercourse if active and satisfaction, painful intercourse
G. Multiple partners, homosexual experience if any
H. Birth control used and effectiveness
I. Ability to carry out role functions to satisfaction
J. Tenderness, pain, discharge of breasts
K. Frequency of breast exams (self and other), Pap smears
L. Number of pregnancies, children
M. Age at menarche, frequency, duration, regularity of periods and amount of menses, dysmenorrhea, bleeding between periods, LMP
N. Date or age at menopause, hot flashes, bleeding or other symptoms
O. Customary medications taken for contraception, infection, estrogen therapy (prescribed and OTC)
P. Past VDRL, mammography, CBC, urinalysis, and other tests and results

### II. Interview and investigate for and record present history:
A. Chief complaint
B. Onset and length of illness
C. S&S presented
D. Knowledge of disease, procedures, and planned therapy
E. Medications taken for reproductive system condition

F. Treatments such as urinary catheter, etc.

G. Results of blood, urine, radiological procedures done

## III. Inspection for:

A. Inflammation, ulceration, discharge, swelling, redness of external genitalia

B. Infestation of pediculosis pubis

C. Bulging of the vaginal walls

D. Color, position, ulcerations, bleeding, discharge, masses of cervix

E. Color, inflammation, ulcers, masses of vaginal mucosa

F. Size, symmetry, contour, moles, dimpling, rash on breasts

G. Color, edema, venous pattern of breasts

H. Size, shape, discharge, rash, ulcers of nipples

## IV. Palpation for:

A. Muscle tone, nodules, or tenderness of vagina

B. Position, shape, mobility, consistency, tenderness of cervix

C. Size, shape, consistency, mobility, tenderness, or masses of uterus

D. Adnexa for tenderness, masses

E. Elasticity, fullness, tenderness, nodularity of both breasts

F. Elasticity, discharge of nipples

G. Axillary areas for enlarged nodes

H. Masses in breast tissue, noting size, shape, location, consistency, tenderness, mobility

# ■ Male Reproductive System Assessment

**DEFINITION:** The collection of a data base concerning the male reproductive system and its functional capabilities to be used in identifying nursing problems related to sexuality, reproduction and elimination

## INTERVENTION

### I. Interview and investigate for and record past history:

A. Previous reproductive system conditions such as venereal diseases, hernia, kidney stones, prostatitis, epididymitis, hydrocele

B. Previous surgeries such as circumcision, herniorrhapy, prostatectomy, orchiectomy

C. Any sores on penis, discharge from penis, pain or masses in testes, scrotal pain or swelling, rashes or irritations of perineal area

D. Difficulty starting or stopping of urination, urgency or frequency of urination, burning or pain on urination, weak urinary stream, incontinence of urine

E. Infertility problem, sexual difficulties, libido

F. Frequency of intercourse if sexually active, multiple partners, ⁻homosexual experiences if any

G. Birth control used, number of children

H. Ability to carry out role functions to satisfaction

I. Customary medications taken for venereal disease, inflammatory conditions of reproductive tract (prescribed and OTC)

J. Past VDRL, x-ray, CBC, urinalysis, and other tests and results

### II. Interview and investigate for and record present history:

A. Chief complaint

B. Onset and length of illness

C. Signs and symptoms presented

D. Knowledge of disease, procedures, and planned therapy

E. Medications taken for any reproductive system problems

F. Treatments such as urinary catheter, etc.

G. Results of blood, urine, radiological studies, and other procedures done

### III. Inspection for:

A. Ulcers, scars, rash, nodules, discharge, swelling of penis, meatus, scrotum

B. Circumcision and cleanliness

C. Infestation and pediculosis pubis

D. Urethal meatus positioned correctly

E. Size and shape of penis and if appropriate for age

F. Contour of scrotum, testes descended

G. Breasts and nipples for symmetry, induration, lesion, drainage

## IV. Palpation for:

A. Masses, tenderness, induration of penal shaft

B. Size, shape, consistency, tenderness, symmetry of testes

C. Spermatic cord and vas deferens and its course

D. Soft, with no swelling or tenderness of prostate by rectal exam

E. Hernia by way of inguinal canal

F. Masses, tenderness, discharge of breasts or nipples

# ■ Abdominal Hysterectomy/Bilateral Salpingo-Oophorectomy

**DEFINITION:** The surgical removal of the uterus, cervix, both fallopian tubes, and both ovaries through an abdominal incision

**CONCEPT/NEED:** Anxiety

**NURSING DIAGNOSIS:** Anxiety related to loss of childbearing potential

**GOAL:** Anxiety will be reduced as evidenced by: verbalization, VS WNL, PERL

| INTERVENTION | RATIONALE |
|---|---|
| **II. Assess for:** | |
| A. Verbal and nonverbal clues to anxiety | A. Patient may be unable to express appropriate feelings in usual manner |
| B. Level of knowledge about procedure/condition | B. Complete information condition/procedure reduces fear and anxiety |
| C. Verbal and nonverbal clues to problems with sexuality | C. Onset of climacteric, reaction to becoming sterile, loss of vaginal sensation |
| D. Clues to hormonal imbalance | D. Depression, elevated emotional sensitivity |
| **III. Administer:** | |
| A. Estrogen therapy as ordered | A. Combats effects of surgically induced menopause |
| B. Tranquilizers as ordered | B. ↓ fear/anxiety |
| **IV. Provide/Perform:** | |
| A. Atmosphere for listening to patient verbalize fears/anxiety | A. Nurse's interest and concern in patient's progress |
| B. Complete information about what may be expected after procedure | B. Assists in relieving fear and anxiety about procedure |

C. Explanation that abdominal cramps and loss of vaginal sensation and secondary sex characteristics will subside, and normal intercourse may be resumed as ordered

C. Assists in relieving fear of impaired sexuality

## V. Teach patient/family:

A. Need for understanding about patient's increased sensitivity or depression

A. Aids in patient's recovery and provides needed reassurance

B. About procedure

B. Complete information dispels myths of procedure

C. About medication

C. Avoids complication

---

**CONCEPT/NEED:** Pain

**NURSING DIAGNOSIS:** Alteration in comfort: pain related to trauma

**GOAL:** Increased comfort as evidenced by: verbalization, decreased request for analgesics

## INTERVENTION

## RATIONALE

### II. Assess for:

A. Characteristics location and extent of pain

A. Complete knowledge of pain aids in proper pain management

B. Abdominal distention

B. Due to surgical trauma

C. Tone of abdominal muscles

C. Excision of large tumor could produce relaxation of abdominal walls

D. Bladder distention

D. Due to edema from surgery

### III. Administer:

A. Analgesics as ordered

A. Pain relief

### IV. Provide/Perform:

A. Pain relief measures as ordered

A. ↓ pain

B. Catheterize as ordered, with proper catheter care

B. Relieves pressure

C. Pass NG as ordered

D. Proper body alignment (See Post-Operative Care, p. 17)

E. Rectal tube as ordered

F. Heat to abdomen as ordered

G. Abdominal binder as ordered

C. Relieves distention

D. Promotes comfort. Aids healing

E. Relieves abdominal distention

F. ↑ peristalsis

G. Supports relaxed abdominal walls

## V. Teach patient/family:

A. Level of discomfort to expect

B. About medication

A. Prepared patient for post-op

B. Avoids complication

---

**CONCEPT/NEED:** Fluid/Electrolyte balance

**NURSING DIAGNOSIS:** Fluid volume deficit related to decreased urinary output

**GOAL:** Adequate fluid volume as evidenced by: good skin turgor, urinary output of 30–50 cc/hr

## INTERVENTION

## RATIONALE

### I. Monitor, describe, record:

A. TPR, BP q 4 hr, peripheral pulses

B. I&O q 4 hr as needed

C. Lab results of electrolytes

A. Insures proper oxygenation, circulation, monitors for signs of infection, hemorrhage

B. Assesses for fluid imbalance or elimination problem

C. Early detection of electrolyte imbalance

### II. Assess for:

A. Urinary retention

B. Adequate intake fluids, (3000 ml/day)

C. Drainage, edema, or redness

D. Constipation, warmth, excess bledding at incisional site

A. From surgical trauma

B. Assists in avoidance of fluid imbalance

C. Signs of infection

D. Presence of complications

|  | E. Vaginal bleeding | E. Sign of hemorrhage |

**III. Administer:**
A. Parenteral fluids as ordered

A. For electrolyte imbalance, volume expanders

**IV. Perform/Provide:**
A. Catheterization as ordered
B. Fluids > 3000 ml/day
C. Inspection of dressing q 24 hr
(See Post-Operative Care, p. 17)

A. Relieves bladder distention
B. Combats fluid imbalance
C. Assesses for hemorrhage or signs of infection

# ■ Abortion

**DEFINITION:** The expulsion of the products of conception. May be induced or spontaneous. Before the fourteenth week of pregnancy, abortion accomplished by D&C or dilation and evacuation. After 14 weeks of pregnancy, abortion accomplished by saline or prostaglandin infusion or injection

**CONCEPT/NEED:** Anxiety

**NURSING DIAGNOSIS:** Anxiety related to unknown

**GOAL:** Reduced anxiety as evidenced by: verbalization, VS WNL

| INTERVENTION | RATIONALE |
|---|---|
| **II. Assess for:** | |
| A. Verbal or nonverbal clues to anxiety or fear | A. Patient may be unable to express feelings in usual manner |
| B. Level of knowledge about condition/procedure | B. Complete information about procedure/condition |
| C. Religious preference or beliefs | C. Appropriate spiritual intervention will aid in recovery and mobilization of additional coping |
| **III. Administer:** | |
| A. Tranquilizers as ordered | A. Combats anxiety |
| **IV. Perform/Provide:** | |
| A. Atmosphere for listening to patient's verbalized fears/anxiety | A. Nurse's interest and concern contributes to patient's progress |
| B. Complete information on procedure/condition | B. Assists in relieving anxiety/fear |
| C. Visits from appropriate clergy as desired | C. Deals with grief and moral implications |
| D. Appropriate sexual counseling if necessary | D. Professional intervention may be indicated |

## V. Teach patient/family:
A. Provide emotional support to patient     A. Helps resolve grieving process satisfactorily

---

**CONCEPT/NEED:** Pain

**NURSING DIAGNOSIS:** Alteration in comfort: pain related to trauma

**GOAL:** Increased comfort as evidenced by: verbalization, lack of grimacing

| INTERVENTION | RATIONALE |
|---|---|
| **II. Monitor, describe, record** | |
| A. TPR, BP q 2 hr | A. Early detection of hemorrhage/infection |
| **II. Assess for:** | |
| A. Characteristics, location, extent of pain | A. Aids in effective pain management |
| B. Nausea/vomiting, severe uterine cramping | B. S&S of infection, hemorrhage |
| **III. Administer:** | |
| A. Analgesics as ordered | A. Pain relief |
| **IV. Provide/Perform:** | |
| A. Pain management as ordered | A. ↓ pain |
| B. Provide emotional support | B. Aids in comfort |

# ■ Dilation and Curettage/ Conization of Cervix

**DEFINITION:** D&C is the widening of the cervical os with dilators and scraping the uterine lining with a curette. Conization of the cervix is the surgical removal of tissue from the cervix for examination or treatment of a cervical condition

**CONCEPT/NEED:** Anxiety

**NURSING DIAGNOSIS:** Anxiety related to trauma, impending surgery

**GOAL:** Anxiety reduced as evidenced by: verbalization, VS WNL

| INTERVENTION | RATIONALE |
|---|---|
| **II. Assess for:** | |
| A. Verbal/nonverbal clues to anxiety/fear | A. Patient may be unable to express feelings in usual manner |
| B. Level of knowledge about procedure | B. Complete information reduces fear/anxiety |
| **III. Administer:** | |
| A. Tranquilizers as ordered | A. Combats anxiety |
| **V. Teach patient/family:** | |
| A. Complete information about procedure | A. Assists in relieving anxiety and fear |
| B. Explanation that procedure will not interfere with sexual activity or childbearing | B. Relieves fear and anxiety |

**CONCEPT/NEED:** Pain

**NURSING DIAGNOSIS:** Alteration in comfort: pain related to trauma

**GOAL:** Increased comfort as evidenced by: verbalization, lack of grimacing

## INTERVENTION

**I. Monitor, describe, record:**
  A. Characteristics of pain

**II. Assess for:**
  A. Characteristics, location and extent of pain; pelvic, low back pain

**III. Administer:**
  A. Analgesics as ordered

**IV. Provide/Perform:**
  A. Pain management as ordered

## RATIONALE

A. Needed for data base

A. Aids in effective pain management

A. Pain relief (cramping)

A. Pain relief

# ■ Radical Mastectomy/ Simple Mastectomy

**DEFINITION:** Radical mastectomy is the surgical removal of a whole breast with the pectoral muscle, lymph nodes of the axilla, and pectoral fascia. A modified radical would not include the pectoral muscle and fascia. Simple mastectomy is the surgical removal of a whole breast

**CONCEPT/NEED:** Anxiety

**NURSING DIAGNOSIS:** Anxiety related to surgery, self image

**GOAL:** Reduced anxiety as evidenced by: verbalization, VS WNL

| INTERVENTION | RATIONALE |
|---|---|
| **II. Assess for:** | |
| A. Verbal/nonverbal clues to anxiety | A. Patient may be unable to communicate feelings in usual manner |
| B. Patient's level of knowledge about condition/procedure, possible outcome | B. Lack of accurate information increases fear/anxiety |
| C. Verbal/nonverbal clues to problems, perceived or real, with sexuality, self-image | C. Procedure is threat to patient's femininity |
| D. Husband's/family's level of knowledge of condition/procedure | D. Husband's/family's support vital to relieving patient's fear/anxiety |
| E. Knowledge of patient/family of outside support organizations | E. Assists in relieving fear/anxiety, provides additional information |
| **III. Administer:** | |
| A. Tranquilizers as ordered | A. ↓ anxiety |
| **IV. Provide/Perform:** | |
| A. Complete accurate information about condition/procedure avoiding false reassurance | A. ↓ anxiety |

B. Proper preparation for husband/family
C. Information on alternate support groups (Reach to Recovery, Inc.)
D. Emotional support
E. Access to spiritual support

B. Effective emotional support, fear/anxiety reduction
C. Additional support promotes anxiety reduction

D. ↓ anxiety
E. ↓ anxiety

V. **Teach patient/family:**
A. Importance of emotional support
B. Importance of planning for future
C. Importance of discussing loss of breast
D. About availability of proper prosthesis

A. ↓ anxiety

B. Anticipating additional surgery/complications
C. Prevents denial/anxiety

D. Can resume pre-op dressing patterns fashionably

---

**CONCEPT/NEED:** Pain

**NURSING DIAGNOSIS:** Alteration in comfort: pain related to incision

**GOAL:** Discomfort will decrease as evidenced by: verbalization, decrease in swelling, no grimacing

## INTERVENTION

## RATIONALE

II. **Assess for:**
A. Proper body alignment
B. Interference of dressing binder with lung expansion
C. Characteristics, location and extent of pain

A. Aids in comfort of pain reduction
B. ↑ comfort/ventilation

C. Effective pain management

III. **Administer:**
A. Analgesics as ordered

A. Pain management

IV. **Perform/Provide:**
A. Proper body alignment/position for comfort

A. ↑ comfort, pain reduction

B. Accurate pain assessment
   (See Post-Operative Care, p.
   17)

B. Needed for data base

C. Elevation for affected arm,
   but not adduction

C. Pain relief, ↑ comfort, proper
   drainage to prevent lymphedema

**V. Teach patient/family:**
   A. Pain will occur and to report
      pain and discomfort

A. Effective pain management

---

**CONCEPT/NEED:** Transport/Circulation

**NURSING DIAGNOSIS:** Alteration in cardiac output: decrease related to
blood loss

**GOAL:** Adequate cardiac output as evidenced by: VS WNL, absence of
bleeding

### INTERVENTION

### RATIONALE

**I. Monitor, describe, record:**
   A. TPR, BP with peripheral
      pulses/BP on unaffected arm

A. Early detection of hemorrhage,
   circulatory problem, infection,
   interference with lung expansion
   by dressing

   B. I&O

B. Early detection of hemorrhage

**II. Assess for:**
   A. Hemovac or sump drain pa-
      tency and type of drainage
      (See Post-Operative Care, p.
      17)

A. Insures proper drainage

**III. Administer:**
   A. Parenteral fluids as ordered

A. Replacement, for blood loss

**IV. Perform/Provide:**
   A. Adequate fluids > 3000
      ml/day
      (See Post-Operative Care, p.
      17)

A. Replace fluids for blood loss

## V. Teach patient/family:

A. Never to have blood drawn, IV started, or BP taken on affected arm

A. Circulation is impaired

# ■ Pelvic Inflammatory Disease

**DEFINITION:** An infection of the pelvic cavity which may or may not involve the ovaries and fallopian tubes. May be chronic or acute and can lead to sterility

**CONCEPT/NEED:** Anxiety

**NURSING DIAGNOSIS:** Anxiety related to sterility

**GOAL:** Reduced anxiety as evidenced by: verbalization, VS WNL

## INTERVENTION

II. **Assess for:**
   A. Verbal and nonverbal clues to anxiety
   B. Level of knowledge about condition
   C. Verbal and nonverbal clues to problems with sexuality

III. **Administer:**
   A. Tranquilizers as ordered

IV. **Provide/Perform:**
   A. Atmosphere for listening to patient's verbalized fear/anxiety
   B. Complete information about condition and treatment
   C. Emotional support

## RATIONALE

A. Patient may be unable to express feelings in usual manner
B. Complete information about condition reduces fear and anxiety
C. Reaction to potential sterility

A. Combats fear/anxiety

A. Nurse's interest, concern contributes to patient's progress
B. Assists in relieving fear/anxiety
C. Helps deal with guilt feelings

---

**CONCEPT/NEED:** Inflammation/Infection

**NURSING DIAGNOSIS:** Potential infection related to contamination

**GOAL:** Absence of infection as evidenced by: temperature WNL, WBC WNL

| **INTERVENTION** | **RATIONALE** |
|---|---|
| **I. Monitor, describe, record:** | |
| A. TPR, BP q 4 hr | A. Early detection of infection |
| B. Vaginal discharge (purulent, malodorous) | B. Indicative of infection |
| C. Lab results | C. Leukocytosis indicative of infection |
| **II. Assess for:** | |
| A. Elevated temperature | A. Indicative of infection |
| B. Characteristics, location and extent of pain | B. Abdominal, pelvic low back pain, acute, sharp is indicative of PID |
| C. Vaginal discharge | C. Indicative of infection |
| D. Nausea, vomiting, malaise, general aching | D. May be indicative of PID |
| E. History of VD or IUD | E. Both may be related to PID |
| **III. Administer:** | |
| A. Antibiotics as ordered | A. Combats infection |
| B. Antipyretics as ordered | B. For fever |
| C. Warm douches as ordered | C. Promotes comfort |
| D. Bedrest as ordered | D. Avoids fatigue |
| E. Abdominal heat as ordered | E. Promotes circulation |
| **IV. Perform/Provide:** | |
| A. Semi-Fowler's position | A. Facilitates drainage |
| B. Perineal care q 3 hr PRN | B. Avoids reinfection |
| C. Adequate fluids > 3000 cc/day | C. For fever and proper fluid balance |
| **V. Teach patient/family:** | |
| A. S&S of complications or re-infection | A. Early detection and treatment |
| B. About alternate methods of birth control if IUD was involved | B. IUD may have caused disease |
| C. Counseling on VD if indicated | C. Prevents reinfection |
| D. About all medications | D. Prevents complications and promotes effective treatment |

# ■ Prostatectomy/Transurethral/ Suprapubic/Retropubic

**DEFINITION:** The surgical removal of part or total prostate gland through the urethra as in the transurethral, through the bladder as in the suprapubic, or through the lower abdomen as in the retropubic

**CONCEPT/NEED:** Anxiety

**NURSING DIAGNOSIS:** Anxiety related to surgery

**GOAL:** Reduced anxiety as evidenced by: verbalization, VS WNL

| INTERVENTION | RATIONALE |
|---|---|
| **II. Assess for:** | |
| A. Verbal and nonverbal clues to anxiety | A. Patient may be unable to express feelings in usual manner |
| B. Level of knowledge about procedure | B. Inaccurate or incomplete knowledge of condition/procedure increases anxiety |
| C. Verbal and nonverbal clues to problems with sexuality | C. Sexual role threatened, radical prostatic surgery can lead to impotence |
| **III. Administer:** | |
| A. Tranquilizers as ordered | A. For anxiety relief |
| **IV. Perform/Provide:** | |
| A. Listening environment for patient | A. ↓ anxiety |
| B. Complete information about procedure/condition and expected outcome | B. Complete, accurate information about condition/procedure aids in anxiety reduction |
| C. Emotional support acceptance | C. Assists in overcoming depression/withdrawal from altered body image/role function |

## V. Teach patient/family:

| | |
|---|---|
| A. About procedure and expected outcome | A. ↓ anxiety |
| B. Visit patient, demonstrate ongoing interest, support | B. Patient may be rendered impotent, needs continued acceptance |
| C. Prosthetic measures such as silicone penis implants are available | C. Permits patient to achieve sex role satisfaction |
| D. In most cases, sexual activity can continue normally in 6–8 weeks | D. Prostatectomy usually does not lead to impotence, only when a radical prostatectomy is done, where pudendal nerves are damaged |

---

**CONCEPT/NEED:** Pain

**NURSING DIAGNOSIS:** Alteration in comfort: pain related to incision

**GOAL:** Increased comfort as evidenced by: verbalization, lack of grimacing

## INTERVENTION

## RATIONALE

**II. Assess for:**

| | |
|---|---|
| A. Characteristics, location and extent of pain | A. Exact knowledge of pain aids in effective pain management |
| B. Presence of bladder spasms | B. Increased pain discomfort, may lead to bleeding |
| C. Catheter patency | C. Obstruction leads to retention, discomfort, other complications |
| D. Type and number of bowel movements | D. Keep soft to prevent straining which leads to discomfort and other complications |
| E. Patterns of post-op ambulation (See Post-Operative Care, p. 17) | E. Should not sit for prolonged period, increases intra-abdominal pressure and discomfort. Chance for bleeding |

**III. Administer:**

| | |
|---|---|
| A. Analgesics as ordered after checking catheter for obstruction | A. Pain reduction and control |
| B. Laxatives as ordered | B. Reduces constipation |

## IV. Perform/Provide:

| | |
|---|---|
| A. Catheter care, bladder irrigations as ordered | A. ↑ comfort, pain reduction |
| B. Instructions for proper body alignment (See Post-Operative Care, p. 17) | B. ↑ comfort and safety, aids in healing, pain reduction |

## V. Teach patient/family:

| | |
|---|---|
| A. Need to avoid constipation (See Post-Operative Care, p. 17) | A. ↑ safety and comfort, pain reduction |

---

**CONCEPT/NEED:** Fluid balance

**NURSING DIAGNOSIS:** Fluid volume deficit related to increased urinary output

**GOAL:** Fluid balance as evidenced by: absence of edema, absence of bladder distention

| INTERVENTION | RATIONALE |
|---|---|
| **I. Monitor, describe, record:** | |
| A. I&O q 4 hr as needed | A. Early detection of obstructed catheter, fluid imbalance |
| **II. Assess for:** | |
| A. Character and flow of urine through catheter line | A. Obstructed catheter line leads to bladder distention, pain, discomfort, bleeding |
| B. Adequate fluid intake | B. Assists in bladder drainage, overall hydration |
| **IV. Perform/Provide:** | |
| A. Bladder irrigations as ordered | A. Insures catheter patency |
| B. Adequate bedside fluids >3000 cc/day | B. Insures hydration and assists in bladder flushing |
| C. Ready access to urinal after catheter is removed | C. Comfort, safety. Urgency may result |

| | |
|---|---|
| D. Major fluid intake in day-time | D. Avoid discomfort at night, nocturia |
| E. Emotional support | E. Assists with fears of incontinence |

**V. Teach patient/family:**

| | |
|---|---|
| A. Importance of not disconnecting or pulling out catheter | A. Safety, prevents injury, maintains proper drainage |
| B. Perineal exercises, tense perineal muscles, hold, relax ×20/hour | B. Regains urinary control |
| C. Keep urine collection bag below bladder level | C. Avoids contamination and discomfort. Possible fluid imbalance |
| D. Protective devices are available to keep dry if problem with incontinence | D. Comfort, self-image |
| E. Importance of adequate fluids | E. Needed for fluid balance |

---

**CONCEPT/NEED:** Inflammation/Infection

**NURSING DIAGNOSIS:** Potential infection related to contamination

**GOAL:** Absence of infection as evidenced by: temperature WNL, drainage clear, area around meatus clean and dry

### INTERVENTION

### RATIONALE

**I. Monitor, describe, record:**

| | |
|---|---|
| A. Temperature q 4 hr (See Post-Operative Care, p. 17) | A. Symptom of infection |

**II. Assess for:**

| | |
|---|---|
| A. Signs of drainage/hemorrhage from incision/catheter drainage | A. Early detection and treatment of hemorrhage/infection |
| B. Irritation/inflammation around meatus related to catheter | B. Meatus may become inflamed or infected from catheter irritation |

**III. Administer:**
   A. Antibiotic as ordered

A. For infection

**IV. Perform/Provide:**
   A. Sitz baths as ordered
   B. Explanation that after cathe-
      ter removal urinary leakage
      and incontinence may occur
      for a time

   C. Aseptic dressing and cath-
      eter care
      (See Post-Operative Care, p.
      17)

A. Promotes healing
B. Relieves anxiety over altered life
   style

C. Promotes urinary flow, prevents
   infection

**V. Teach patient/family:**
   A. S&S to be alert for such as
      drainage or intermittent
      hematuria. After 2–4 wks,
      bleeding, signs of infection

A. Early detection of complications

# ■ Prostatic Hypertrophy/Prostatitis

**DEFINITION:** Prostatic hypertrophy is an enlargement of the prostate gland resulting in partial or complete obstruction of urination or incomplete emptying of the bladder. Prostatitis is the inflammation of the prostate gland causing frequency, urgency, and pain on urination

**CONCEPT/NEED:** Inflammation/Infection

**NURSING DIAGNOSIS:** Potential infection related to urinary retention

**GOAL:** Absence of infection as evidenced by: temperature WNL, absence of bacteria in urine

### INTERVENTION

### RATIONALE

I. **Monitor, describe, record:**
   A. TPR, BP q 4 hr

   B. I&O q 8 hr

A. Early detection of inflammation, infection

B. Early detection of fluid imbalance/urinary retention/urine stasis

II. **Assess for:**
   A. Hesitancy, stream, force of urine
   B. Urgency, frequency, nocturia, dysuria, hematuria
   C. Proper fluid intake
   D. Proper catheter drainage if indicated
   E. Level of knowledge of probable procedures, cystoscopy, massage, etc

A. Indicative of BPH or prostatitis/obstruction
B. S&S of condition

C. Insures hydration
D. Prevents obstruction, infection

E. Relieves anxiety, enhances co-operation

III. **Administer:**
   A. Antibiotics as ordered
   B. Prostatic massage as ordered
   C. Antispasmodics and bladder sedatives as ordered

A. For infection
B. For diagnostic test, specimen
C. Bladder irritability

D. Stool softeners as ordered     D. ↑ comfort, ↓ pain

E. Analgesics as ordered        E. Pain management

## IV. Perform/Provide:

A. Adequate fluids > 3000 ml/day but do not force fluids
     A. Promotes drainage, prevents complication of dehydration

B. Ready access to urinal       B. Comfort/safety

C. Proper catheter care BID if indicated
     C. Infection prevention

## V. Teach patient/family:

A. Finish medication         A. Insures proper antibiotic levels

B. Not to FF               B. Must maintain adequate drug levels in urine

C. Avoid foods or drink with diuretic action, e.g., coffee, tea, cola, chocolate, spices
     C. Must maintain adequate drug levels in urine

D. Avoid intercourse during inflammation
     D. Infection may be transmitted resulting in reinfection

E. Avoid sitting for prolonged periods
     E. Irritating

F. Importance of follow-up exam
     F. Chronic nature of condition

G. Not to delay urination      G. Prevents urinary stasis/retention

H. S&S of complications       H. Early detection and treatment

# ■ Tubal Ligation/Tubal Pregnancy

**DEFINITION:** Tubal ligation is a surgical procedure in which sterilization is attained by interrupting the passage of the ova through the fallopian tubes. This may be done through an abdominal incision in which the tubes are tied and then cut or through laparoscopy in which the tubes are sealed or electrocoagulated. Tubal pregnancy is the implantation of a pregnancy in a fallopian tube. This condition is corrected by a salpingectomy, the surgical removal of the fallopian tube

**CONCEPT/NEED:** Anxiety

**NURSING DIAGNOSIS:** Anxiety related to surgery

**GOAL:** Reduced anxiety as evidenced by: verbalization, pulse WNL

| INTERVENTION | RATIONALE |
|---|---|
| **II. Assess for:** | |
| A. Verbal and nonverbal clues to anxiety/fear | A. Client may be unable to express appropriate feelings in usual manner |
| B. Level of knowledge about procedure | B. Complete information about procedure reduces fear and anxiety |
| C. Verbal and nonverbal clues to problems with sexuality | C. Feelings of loss in sexuality or body image can result from tubal ligation |
| **III. Administer:** | |
| A. Tranquilizers as ordered | A. Relieves anxiety |
| **IV. Perform/Provide:** | |
| A. Atmosphere for listening to client's verbalized fears/anxiety | A. Nurse's interest and concern contributes to patient's progress |
| B. Complete information about procedure and expected outcome | B. Assists in relieving fear/anxiety |
| C. Emotional support | C. Assists in coping with feeling of loss in sexuality/body image |

## V. Teach patient/family:
A. In tubal ligation, pregnancy is not possible

A. Assists in anxiety and fear reduction

B. Procedure is generally not reversible

B. Assists in anxiety and fear reduction

C. Sexual drive is not affected by procedure

C. Assists in anxiety and fear reduction

---

**CONCEPT/NEED:** Comfort

**NURSING DIAGNOSIS:** Alteration in comfort: pain related to trauma of surgery

**GOAL:** Minimal or absence of pain as evidenced by: verbalization, diminished need for pain medication

## INTERVENTION

## RATIONALE

### II. Assess for:
A. Characteristics, location and extent of pain

A. Aids in proper effective pain management. Also is diagnostic for complication of tubal pregnancy

B. Severe lower abdominal pain with vaginal bleeding

B. Indicative of ruptured tube

C. Abdominal distention/urinary retention
(See Post-Operative Care, p. 17)

C. From surgical trauma

### III. Administer:
A. Analgesics as ordered

A. Pain management

### IV. Perform/Provide:
A. Pain management as ordered
B. Catheterization as ordered
C. Pass rectal tube as ordered
(See Post-Operative Care, p. 17)

A. Promotes comfort
B. Relieves distention
C. Relieves gas

# ■ Vaginal Hysterectomy/Anterior and Posterior Colporrhaphy

**DEFINITION:** Vaginal hysterectomy is the surgical removal of the uterus through the vagina. Anterior and/or posterior colporrhaphy is the surgical repair of a cystocele (bladder protruding down into the bladder) or rectocele (rectal protruding up into the vagina)

**CONCEPT/NEED:** Anxiety

**NURSING DIAGNOSIS:** Anxiety related to surgery

**GOAL:** Decreased anxiety as evidenced by: verbalization, pulse WNL

| INTERVENTION | RATIONALE |
|---|---|
| **II. Assess for:** | |
| A. Verbal and nonverbal clues to anxiety | A. Patient may be unable to express appropriate feelings in usual manner |
| B. Level of knowledge about procedure/condition | B. Complete information about condition/procedure reduces fear/anxiety |
| C. Verbal and nonverbal clues to problems with sexuality | C. Reaction to becoming sterile, loss of vaginal sensation |
| **III. Administer:** | |
| A. Tranquilizers as ordered | A. ↓ fear/anxiety |
| **IV. Perform/Provide:** | |
| A. Atmosphere for listening to patient's verbalized fears/anxiety | A. Nurse's interest and concern contributes to patient's progress |
| B. Complete information on procedure/condition, what may be expected after procedure | B. Assists in relieving fear and anxiety |
| C. Explanation that loss of vaginal sensation will subside and normal intercourse may be resumed as ordered | C. Assists in relieving fear and anxiety of impaired sexuality |

## V. Teach patient/family:

| | |
|---|---|
| A. About cessation of menstruation | A. Relieves fear/anxiety |
| B. Need for assistance in dealing with perceived change in body image | B. Relieves fear/anxiety, promotes rapid recovery |

---

**CONCEPT/NEED:** Infection

**NURSING DIAGNOSIS:** Potential infection related to contamination

**GOAL:** Absence of infection as evidenced by: absence of foul smelling discharge, temperature WNL

## INTERVENTION

## RATIONALE

### I. Monitor, describe, record:
A. TPR, q 2 hr

A. Assess for S&S of infection

### III. Administer:
A. Catheterization as ordered

A. Relieves retention

B. Antibiotics as ordered

B. For infection (surgical or bladder)

### IV. Perform/Provide:
A. Catheter care BID, PRN

A. ↓ infection

B. Perineal care after each elimination

B. ↓ infection

C. Proper body alignment

C. ↑ comfort/healing

### V. Teach patient/family:
A. Avoid tub baths, coitus, or douching as ordered

A. Infection prevention

B. S&S of infection

B. Early detection and treatment

C. Perineal hygiene
(See Post-Operative Care, p. 17)

C. Prevents infection

# EYE, EAR, NOSE, THROAT SYSTEM STANDARDS

- Eye, Ear, Nose, Throat System Assessment
- Cataract Removal
- Corneal Transplant
- Deviated Nasal Septum/Submucous Resection
- Enucleation/Evisceration
- Glaucoma/Iridectomy
- Meniere's Syndrome
- Retinal Detachment
- Stapedectomy
- Tonsillectomy/Adenoidectomy

# ■ Eye, Ear, Nose, Throat System Assessment

**DEFINITION:** The collection of a data base concerning the eye, ear, nose, throat system and its functional capabilities to be used in identifying nursing problems related to sensory perception and sensory deprivation

## INTERVENTION

### I. Interview and investigate for and record past history:
A. Previous conditions such as glaucoma, cataract, conjunctivitis, retinal detachment, hypertension, diabetes, otitis media, otosclerosis, tonsillitis, deviated septum, rhinitis
B. Previous surgeries such as tonsillectomy, cataract, corneal, retinal, stapedectomy, mastoidectomy, submucous resection, plastic surgery
C. Any blurred or doubled vision, spots, or visual changes such as flashes, light halos, pain, burning, itching, discharge, swelling of eyes, night blindness or color blindness, tinnitus, buzzing, pain, itching, drainage of eyes, loss of equilibrium, vertigo, headaches, pain or stiffness in neck, throat pain or difficulty swallowing, stuffy, runny nose, nose bleeds, hoarseness, soreness in mouth, tongue, or gums
D. Sight impairment and use of glasses or contact lenses, hearing impairment and use of hearing aid or lip reading, impairment in sense of smell, taste, loss of teeth, and use of partial or full dentures
E. Last visit to dentist, physician for vision and hearing testing
F. Allergies to pollens, other environmental pollutants
G. Care of glasses, contacts, hearing aid, dentures, eye prosthesis
H. Response to noise levels, use of hairspray, Q-tips to clean ears
I. Use of medications (prescribed and OTC)
J. Effect of impairment on self-concept and occupation
K. Factors affecting impairment such as age, emotions, disease
L. Past x-rays, acuity testing and kind, refraction, or others and results

### II. Interview and investigate for and record present history:
A. Chief complaint
B. Onset and length of illness
C. S&S
D. Knowledge of disease, procedures, and planned therapy

E. Medications taken such as antibiotics, eye or ear drops, nose drops, and others
F. Treatments such as packing, eye dressings, irrigations, special diets
G. Results of blood, urine, radiological exams, and procedures

## III. Inspection for:
A. Symmetry of eyes, lids, brows
B. Visual acuity using Snellen chart
C. Peripheral vision test by confrontation
D. Color, structure, edema, lesions of lids
E. Color of conjunctivas and scleras, note opacities and markings of iris
F. Round, intact lacrimal glands
G. Size, shape, equality, reaction of pupils
H. Intactness of extraocular movements
 I. Red reflex, optic disk, and blood vessels by use of the ophthalmoscope
J. Deformities, lesions of external ear and auricles
K. Color, size and position (symmetry) of the ears and auricles
L. Discharge or inflammation of the canals and drums
M. Color, thickness, light reflex of drums, by use of the otoscope
N. Auditory acuity by whisper test, Weber or Rinne tests
O. Deformities, shape, symmetry, inflammation of nose by use of nasal speculum
P. Color, swelling, drainage, blood of mucosa of nose, the septum for deviation and the turbinates for swelling, color, polyps
Q. Color, ulcers, dryness, cracking, edema of lips
R. Color, swelling, bleeding, inflammation of gums and buccal cavity and throat
S. Soft palate and uvula rising
T. Tonsils if present for size, redness, swelling

## IV. Palpation for:
A. Firmness, masses, elasticity, pain of pinna
B. Tenderness in frontal or maxillary sinuses
C. Structure of nose

# ■ Cataract Removal

**DEFINITION:** The surgical removal of a lens that has matured or become cloudy or opaque causing visual impairment. Causes of cataract formation include degenerative, congenital, trauma, or disease. A lens may be implanted following removal of the cataract if indicated and eliminates the need for post-operative spectacles or contact lenses

**CONCEPT/NEED:** Anxiety/Fear

**NURSING DIAGNOSIS:** Anxiety related to loss of sight

**GOAL:** Decreased anxiety as evidenced by: verbalization, pulse WNL, ability to sleep at night

| INTERVENTION | RATIONALE |
|---|---|
| **II. Assess for:** | |
| A. Verbal and nonverbal clues to anxiety | A. Patient may be unable to express feelings in the usual manner |
| B. Patient's level of knowledge about condition/procedure | B. Knowledge deficit increases anxiety/fear |
| C. Patient's pre-operative degree of vision | C. Vision will initially be impaired in affected eye, post-operatively |
| **III. Administer:** | |
| A. Anti-anxiety medication as ordered | A. ↓ anxiety |
| B. Special glasses or contact lenses as ordered | B. Restores vision in affected eye |
| C. Protective eye shields post-operatively as ordered | C. Prevents injury |
| **IV. Perform/Provide:** | |
| A. Listening atmosphere free of stress-producing distractions for patient to verbalize feelings | A. Anxiety reduction/promotion of communication |

B. Complete information about procedure/condition

B. ↓ anxiety/fear

C. Adequate assessment of pre-operative visual activity

C. Vision will initially be impaired in affected eye, possibly compounding difficulty with degree of vision

D. Emotional support

D. ↓ anxiety/fear

E. Pre-operative orientation with hospital room, surroundings

E. Safety, anxiety reduction post-operative related to decreased degree of vision

F. Diversional activities, e.g., talking books, radio, encourage visitors, etc

F. Combats problem with sensory deprivation

## V. Teach patient/family:

A. Affected eye will be covered after procedure

A. Relieves anxiety over loss of vision

B. If glasses are indicated, post-operative depth perception will be altered

B. Glasses magnify objects 25–30%

C. Glasses will be temporary

C. Allows time for healing to occur, up to 3 months

D. Without glasses, patient will not be able to focus eye

D. ↓ anxiety/fear

E. If contact lenses are indicated, patient will be fitted after 3 months

E. Allows time for healing to occur, up to 3 months

F. With contact lenses patient can focus, but will require glasses for near vision

F. ↓ anxiety/fear

G. With intraocular lens implant, patient will require glasses for near vision, will be able to focus, and not suffer from altered depth perception

G. ↓ anxiety/fear

---

**CONCEPT/NEED:** Pain

**NURSING DIAGNOSIS:** Alteration in comfort: pain related to trauma

**GOAL:** Increased comfort as evidenced by: verbalization, decreased request for pain medications

## INTERVENTION

## RATIONALE

**II. Assess for:**
    A. Characteristics, location and extent of pain
    B. S&S of discomfort

A. Necessary for proper pain management
B. Early detection and correction of condition

**III. Administer:**
    A. Analgesics as ordered
    B. Sedatives/hypnotics as ordered
    C. Atropine drops to eyes as ordered
    D. Antiemetics as ordered. Stool softeners

A. ↓ pain
B. Comfort/rest/sleep
C. Pain reduction
D. ↓ strain and pain related to nausea/vomiting, bowel elimination

**IV. Perform/Provide:**
    A. Firm, low pillow and elevate head of bed 30–45 degrees
    B. Place small pillows under knees and small of back for short periods
    C. Assistance with eating if necessary
    D. Bedrest

A. ↑ comfort, ↓ strain
B. ↑ comfort, relieves strain
C. May need help in identifying foods/opening cartons
D. Avoids strain and fatigue

**V. Teach patient/family:**
    A. Avoid sneezing, coughing, straining as much as possible

A. ↓ pain/strain, ↑ comfort

---

**CONCEPT/NEED:** Infection

**NURSING DIAGNOSIS:** Potential infection related to contamination

**GOAL:** Absence of infection as evidenced by: WBC WNL, temperature WNL, absence of drainage

| INTERVENTION | RATIONALE |
|---|---|
| **I. Monitor, describe, record:** | |
| A. Temperature q 4 hr | A. Early detection of infection |
| B. Dressing for drainage q 1 hr | B. Early detection of infection |
| **II. Assess for:** | |
| A. Excessive pain | A. Symptom of hemorrhage/infection |
| B. S&S of infection | B. Early detection and treatment |
| **III. Administer:** | |
| A. Antibiotics as ordered | A. Combats infection |
| B. Instillation of eye preparations as ordered | B. Infection avoidance |
| **IV. Perform/Provide:** | |
| A. Dressing changes as ordered | A. Infection avoidance |
| B. Protective eye shield as ordered | B. Protection from injury |
| **V. Teach patient/family:** | |
| A. Proper eye care as ordered | A. Safety, compliance of treatment |
| B. S&S of infection | B. Early detection/treatment |
| C. Avoid heavy lifting, stooping, or straining for 1–2 months | C. Prevents re-injury to affected eye |

# ■ Corneal Transplant

**DEFINITION:** The surgical replacement of a damaged cornea with a normal donor eye graft

**CONCEPT/NEED:** Anxiety

**NURSING DIAGNOSIS:** Anxiety related to loss of sight

**GOAL:** Reduction in anxiety as evidenced by: verbalization, pulse WNL, ability to sleep at night

| INTERVENTION | RATIONALE |
|---|---|
| **II. Assess for:** | |
| A. Verbal/nonverbal clues to anxiety/fear | A. Patient may be unable to express feelings in usual manner |
| B. Patient's level of knowledge about condition/procedure | B. Knowledge deficit increases anxiety/fear |
| C. Patient's pre-operative degree of vision | C. Usually poor related to corneal injury |
| **III. Administer:** | |
| A. Anti-anxiety drugs as ordered | A. Anxiety relief |
| **IV. Perform/Provide:** | |
| A. Listening atmosphere free of stress-producing distractions, for patient to verbalize feelings | A. Anxiety/fear reduction, promotion of communication |
| B. Complete information about condition/procedure | B. ↓ fear/anxiety |
| C. Adequate assessment of pre-operative visual activity | C. Aids in post-operative planning |
| D. Orient patient to surroundings pre-operatively | D. Eyes will be covered post-operatively |
| E. Emotional support | E. ↓ fear/anxiety |

| | |
|---|---|
| F. Diversional activities, post-operative, e.g., talking books, radio, encourage visitors | F. Prevents complication of altered sensory perception |

**V. Teach patient/family:**

| | |
|---|---|
| A. Procedure is better than 80% effective in improving vision to affected eye/eyes | A. ↓ anxiety/fear |

---

**CONCEPT/NEED:** Infection

**NURSING DIAGNOSIS:** Potential infection related to contamination

**GOAL:** Absence of infection as evidenced by: temperature WNL, WBC WNL, absence of drainage

**INTERVENTION**

**RATIONALE**

| | |
|---|---|
| **I. Monitor, describe, record:** | |
| A. Temperature q 4 hr | A. Early detection of infection |
| B. Drainage on dressings | B. Early detection of infection |
| **II. Assess for:** | |
| A. S&S of infection | A. Early detection of infection |
| **III. Administer:** | |
| A. Antibiotics as ordered | A. Combats infection |
| B. Topical corticosteroids as ordered | B. Helps prevent tissue rejection |
| C. Instillation of eye preparations as ordered | C. Avoids infection |
| **IV. Perform/Provide:** | |
| A. Sterile dressing changes as ordered | A. Infection avoidance |
| B. Contact lenses as ordered | B. For protection of suture line/infection reduction |
| **V. Teach patient/family:** | |
| A. Importance of avoiding fatigue | A. Aids in proper healing/recovery |

B. Proper eye care as ordered

C. S&S of infection/inflammation

D. Usually eyes will be unpatched on third day

E. Sutures will be removed in 7–8 months

F. Avoid straining, stooping, heavy lifting as ordered

B. ↑ safety, compliance to treatment

C. Early detection and treatment

D. ↓ anxiety

E. Allows for complete healing

F. Prevents complication of straining, constipation avoidance

# ■ Deviated Nasal Septum/ Submucous Resection

**DEFINITION:** Deviated nasal septum is a condition in which the septum is bent or deviated to one side or both sides from the midline

**CONCEPT/NEED:** Oxygenation

**NURSING DIAGNOSIS:** Ineffective breathing pattern related to obstruction

**GOAL:** Adequate breathing pattern as evidenced by: breathing through mouth

## INTERVENTION

I. **Monitor, describe, record:**
   A. TPR, BP (rectal temperature)

II. **Assess for:**
   A. S&S of lack of $O_2$
   B. Proper placement of nasal packing
   C. Respiratory distress

III. **Administer:**
   A. NPO ×6–8 hours as ordered

   B. Ice packs as ordered

IV. **Perform/Provide:**
   A. Tape packing strings to cheeks
   (See Post-Operative Care, p. 17)

V. **Teach patient/family:**
   A. Avoid nose blowing for 4 days

## RATIONALE

A. Early detection and correction of poor oxygenation, circulation

A. Early detection and correction
B. Proper placement necessary to allow oxygenation
C. Edema, bleeding, packing

A. Prevents irritation leading to hemorrhage
B. ↓ bleeding, edema

A. Prevents accidental dislodging of packing

A. Prevention of hemorrhage

B. S&S of complications
C. No stooping or straining (See Post-Operative Care, p. 17)

B. Early detection and correction
C. Prevention of hemorrhage

---

**CONCEPT/NEED:** Pain

**NURSING DIAGNOSIS:** Alteration of comfort: pain related to trauma

**GOAL:** Increased comfort as evidenced by: verbalization, decreased request for pain medications

## INTERVENTION

**II. Assess for:**
    A. Characteristics, location and extent of pain
    B. Verbal, nonverbal clues to discomfort

**III. Administer:**
    A. Analgesics as ordered
    B. Ice packs as ordered

**IV. Perform/Provide:**
    A. Pain assessment
    B. Good oral hygiene q 1–2 hr

    C. Position of comfort as permitted by order

**V. Teach patient/family:**
    A. Good oral hygiene
    B. Proper use of ice packs

## RATIONALE

A. Effective pain management

B. Patient may be unable to convey feeling of discomfort in expected manner

A. Relieves pain
B. Reduces edema, pain relief

A. Proper pain management
B. ↑ comfort (blood taste causes nausea)
C. ↑ comfort

A. ↑ comfort, infection prevention
B. Reduction of edema, discoloration

# ■ Enucleation/Evisceration

**DEFINITION:** Enucleation is the surgical removal of the eyeball as a result of trauma, infection, tumor, or foreign bodies. Evisceration is the surgical scooping out of the contents of the eye

**CONCEPT/NEED:** Anxiety

**NURSING DIAGNOSIS:** Anxiety related to loss of eye

**GOAL:** Reduction in anxiety as evidenced by: verbalization, pulse WNL, ability to sleep at night

| INTERVENTION | RATIONALE |
|---|---|
| **II. Assess for:** | |
| A. Verbal and nonverbal clues to anxiety/fear | A. Patient may be unable to express feelings in usual manner |
| B. Patient's level of knowledge about condition/procedure | B. Knowledge deficit increases fear/anxiety |
| C. Potential problems with self-image related to loss of eye | C. Patient may perceive loss as permanent disfigurement |
| **III. Administer:** | |
| A. Anti-anxiety medication as ordered | A. ↓ anxiety |
| **IV. Perform/Provide:** | |
| A. Listening atmosphere for patient to verbalize feelings | A. ↓ fear/anxiety, promotes communication |
| B. Complete information about condition/procedure | B. ↓ anxiety/fear |
| C. Information about available ability of prosthesis | C. Assists with promotion of self-image |
| D. Emotional support and encouragement | D. Assists with promotion of self-image |
| **V. Teach patient/family:** | |
| A. Prosthesis may be indistinguishable from good eye | A. ↓ fear/anxiety, promotes self-image |

B. Assistance from organization is available depending on degree of vision impairment

B. ↓ fear/anxiety, promotes self-image

---

**CONCEPT/NEED:** Pain

**NURSING DIAGNOSIS:** Alteration in comfort: pain related to trauma

**GOAL:** Increased comfort as evidenced by: verbalization, decreased request for pain medication

### INTERVENTION

### RATIONALE

II. **Assess for:**
   A. Characteristics, location and extent of pain
   B. Verbal and nonverbal clues to discomfort

A. Necessary for proper pain management
B. Early detection and treatment/correction

III. **Administer:**
   A. Analgesics as ordered

A. Pain relief

IV. **Perform/Provide:**
   A. Comfortable position as allowed with proper body alignment

A. ↑ comfort, pain relief

   B. Accurate pain assessment
   C. Quiet, restful environment for patient
   D. Special attention to decreased visual activity, or blindness due to dressing (place things in same place for patient each time, siderail precaution, announce presence, place call bell in hand)

B. Effective pain management
C. ↑ comfort/sleep/rest, avoids complications of fatigue
D. ↑ comfort/safety

---

**CONCEPT/NEED:** Infection

**NURSING DIAGNOSIS:** Potential infection related to contamination

**GOAL:** Absence of infection as evidenced by: temperature WNL, lack of drainage, WBC WNL

| INTERVENTION | RATIONALE |
|---|---|
| **I. Monitor, describe, record:** | |
| A. TPR, BP q 4 hr | A. Early detection of infection/inflammation/hemorrhage |
| **II. Assess for:** | |
| A. S&S of infection | A. Early detection of infection |
| B. Severe headache on operated side (See Post-Operative Care, p. 17) | B. Meningitis occasionally occurs due to thrombosis of adjacent veins |
| **III. Administer:** | |
| A. Antibiotics as ordered | A. Combats infection |
| **IV. Perform/Provide:** | |
| A. (See Post-Operative Care, p. 17) | A. For more information |
| **V. Teach patient/family:** | |
| A. S&S of infection | A. Early detection and treatment |
| B. A prosthetic eye can be used as ordered after 6–8 weeks | B. ↑ self-esteem |
| C. Types of prosthetics available (See Post-Operative Care, p. 17) | C. Identifies possible option for the patient |

# ■ Glaucoma/Iridectomy

**DEFINITION:** Glaucoma is a disease of the eye in which there is a buildup of intraocular tension caused by increased production and decreased excretion of aqueous humor (acute) or the obstruction in the excretion of aqueous humor (chronic). Causes visual impairment and over a period of time blindness. Iridectomy is the surgical procedure performed to relieve pressure by allowing for excretion of aqueous humor

**CONCEPT/NEED:** Sensory perception

**NURSING DIAGNOSIS:** Uncompensated sensory deficit: vision related to inability to identify objects

**GOAL:** Increased vision as evidenced by: instillation of eye drops, absence of progression of disease

| INTERVENTION | RATIONALE |
|---|---|
| **II. Assess for:** | |
| A. Degree and acuity of vision | A. Blurred vision, rainbow around lights will occur in acute condition, peripheral vision impaired |
| **III. Administer:** | |
| A. Miotics as ordered | A. Constrict pupil, ↓ intraocular pressure |
| B. Acetazolamide as ordered | B. ↓ formations of aqueous humor, intraocular pressure |
| C. Fluid restriction as ordered | C. Prevent over-hydration, ↓ intraocular pressure |
| D. Timoloc as ordered | D. Blurred vision, rainbow around lights will occur in acute condition, peripheral vision impaired |
| E. Epinephrine as ordered | E. Blurred vision, rainbow around lights will occur in acute condition, peripheral vision impaired |
| **IV. Perform/Provide:** | |
| A. Assistance depending on degree needed | A. Insures safety |

**CONCEPT/NEED:** Anxiety

**NURSING DIAGNOSIS:** Anxiety related to loss of vision.

**GOAL:** Reduced anxiety as evidenced by: verbalization, ability to sleep at night, pulse WNL

| INTERVENTION | RATIONALE |
|---|---|
| **II. Assess for:** | |
| A. Verbal/nonverbal clues to anxiety | A. Needed to identify anxiety |
| B. Patient's level of knowledge about condition/procedure | B. Knowledge deficit increases anxiety |
| **III. Administer:** | |
| A. Anti-anxiety medication as ordered | A. ↓ anxiety |
| **IV. Perform/Provide:** | |
| A. Listening atmosphere free of stress, producing distractions for patient | A. ↓ anxiety, promotes communication |
| B. Complete information about condition/procedure | B. ↓ fear/anxiety |
| C. Orientation of surroundings | C. ↓ anxiety post-operatively |
| **V. Teach patient/family:** | |
| A. Condition is not reversible but is controllable with strict adherence to medical regimen | A. ↓ anxiety/fear |

**CONCEPT/NEED:** Pain

**NURSING DIAGNOSIS:** Alteration in comfort: pain related to trauma

**GOAL:** Increased comfort as evidenced by: verbalization, reduced request for pain medication

| INTERVENTION | RATIONALE |
|---|---|

**II. Assess for:**

A. Characteristics, location and extent of pain
    A. Effective pain management (headache, severe eye pain)

B. Patterns of rest/sleep
    B. Early detection of problem/early correction

C. Verbal/nonverbal clues to discomfort
    C. Patient may not express discomfort in expected manner

D. Easy access to personal items, call bell, siderail precautions
    D. ↑ safety/comfort

**III. Administer:**

A. Analgesics as ordered
    A. Pain relief

B. Sedatives/hypnotics
    B. Promotes proper rest/sleep patterns

C. Bedrest as ordered
    C. ↑ comfort, ↓ pain

D. Antiemetics as ordered
    D. Prevents discomfort from straining

**IV. Perform/Provide:**

A. Quiet, restful atmosphere free from unnecessary distractions
    A. Promotes rest/sleep/comfort

B. Personal items around bed in same place everytime
    B. Encourages independence, sight impaired due to dressings

C. Emotional support and encouragement of independence
    C. Promotes independence

**V. Teach patient/family:**

A. Pain control measures
    A. ↓ discomfort

# ■ Meniere's Syndrome

**DEFINITION:** A condition of the inner ear as a result of labyrinthine dysfunction causing vertigo, tinnitus, and progressive deafness in the affected ear

**CONCEPT/NEED:** Anxiety

**NURSING DIAGNOSIS:** Anxiety related to possible hearing loss

**GOAL:** Reduction in anxiety as evidenced by: verbalization, pulse WNL, ability to sleep at night

## INTERVENTION

II. **Assess for:**
   - A. Verbal/nonverbal clues to anxiety
   - B. Patient's environmental safety factors
   - C. Degree of vertigo being experienced
   - D. Patient's level of hearing

III. **Administer:**
   - A. Valium IV as ordered
   - B. Dramamine rectal suppository as ordered
   - C. Other antivertigo drugs as ordered
   - D. Vasodilating drugs (Priscoline, Banthine)
   - E. Anti-anxiety drugs as ordered
   - F. Atropine SQ

IV. **Perform/Provide:**
   - A. Safe, obstacle-free environment
   - B. Quiet, distraction-free environment

## RATIONALE

   - A. Patient may be unable to express feelings in the usual manner
   - B. Condition may produce falls related to vertigo resulting in injury
   - C. Degrees vary in severity
   - D. Necessary for proper condition management planning

   - A. Combats vertigo, ↓ anxiety
   - B. Combats vertigo
   - C. Combats vertigo
   - D. ↓ tinnitus
   - E. Combats anxiety
   - F. May terminate attack

   - A. ↓ potential for falls
   - B. ↓ chances for vertigo

C. Assist ambulating

D. Speak softly and directly to patient

E. Give emotional support

F. Complete information about condition/procedure

C. ↑ safety

D. Avoids head-turning agitation

E. Relieves anxiety, encourages cooperation

F. ↓ anxiety

## V. Teach patient/family:

A. Turn on affected side after attack

B. Surgery may be indicated if condition deteriorates progressively

C. Lie down or sit down at onset of vertigo

D. Avoid smoking if possible

E. Avoid fast, jerky movements of head

F. Tinnitus may be continually present

A. ↓ complications of vertigo

B. Conserves hearing

C. ↑ safety by preventing falls

D. Avoids vasospasms and vasoconstriction which could lead to attack

E. Causes vertigo

F. ↓ anxiety

---

**CONCEPT/NEED:** Self-concept

**NURSING DIAGNOSIS:** Disturbance in self concept related to hearing loss

**GOAL:** Increased self-concept as evidenced by: verbalization, ability to perform daily functions

## INTERVENTION

## RATIONALE

### II. Assess for:

A. Verbal/nonverbal clues to altered self-concept

A. Clues may not be overt. Patient may have difficulty expressing feelings in usual manner

### IV. Perform/Provide:

A. Encouragement to follow through with treatment

A. Prevents further hearing loss, promotes self-concept

# ■ Retinal Detachment

**DEFINITION:** A condition in which there is a partial or complete detachment of the retina from the choroid. May be caused by trauma, hemorrhage, tumor, or degeneration. Surgical procedures to correct this condition include photocoagulation, cryopexy, or scleral buckling

**CONCEPT/NEED:** Anxiety

**NURSING DIAGNOSIS:** Anxiety related to loss of vision

**GOAL:** Decreased anxiety as evidenced by: verbalization, pulse WNL, ability to sleep at night

| INTERVENTION | RATIONALE |
|---|---|
| **II. Assess for:** | |
| A. Verbal/nonverbal clues to fear/anxiety | A. Patient may be unable to express feelings in usual manner |
| B. Patient's level of knowledge about condition/procedure | B. Knowledge deficit increases anxiety/fear |
| C. Patient's pre-operative degree of vision | C. Aids in post-operative planning, symptoms "sooty" vision, sudden onset of rapidly progressing blindness |
| **III. Administer:** | |
| A. Anti-anxiety medication as ordered | A. ↓ anxiety/fear, promotion of communication |
| **IV. Perform/Provide:** | |
| A. Listening atmosphere, free from stress-producing distractions for patient | A. ↓ anxiety/fear, promotion of communication |
| B. Complete information about condition/procedure | B. ↓ anxiety/fear |
| C. Adequate assessment of pre-operative visual activity | C. Aids in post-operative planning |
| D. Orient patient to surroundings pre-operatively | D. Eyes will be covered post-operative/anxiety reduction |

E. Emotional support

F. Diversional activities post-operative, e.g., talking books, radio, encourage visitors

**V. Teach patient/family:**

A. Restoring vision acceptability depends on extent and length of detachment before surgery and 90% are cured

E. ↓ anxiety/fear

F. Prevents anxiety/fear complications of altered sensory perception

A. Aids in anxiety/fear reduction

---

**CONCEPT/NEED:** Pain

**NURSING DIAGNOSIS:** Alteration in comfort: pain related to trauma

**GOAL:** Increased comfort as evidenced by: verbalization, absence of grimacing

### INTERVENTION

**II. Assess for:**

A. Characteristics, location and extent of pain

B. S&S of discomfort

**III. Administer:**

A. Analgesics as ordered

**IV. Perform/Provide:**

A. Accurate pain assessment

B. Quiet, restful atmosphere, free from unnecessary distraction

C. Comfortable position with proper body alignment as ordered (will vary depending on extent and location of detachment)

D. Assistance with eating and hygiene

### RATIONALE

A. Necessary for proper pain management

B. Early detection and correction of condition

A. Pain relief

A. Proper pain management

B. Comforts/assists with pain control

C. ↑ comfort, pain control

D. ↑ comfort

## V. Teach patient/family:

| | |
|---|---|
| A. Importance of not straining, e.g., stooping, bending, lifting, constipation | A. Prevents re-injury |
| B. Avoidance of contact sports for life if ordered | B. Prevents re-injury |

---

**CONCEPT:** Sensory perception

**NURSING DIAGNOSIS:** Sensory/Perceptual alteration, deprivation related to lack of vision

**GOAL:** Absence of sensory perceptual alteration as evidenced by: acceptance of diversional activities

### INTERVENTION

### RATIONALE

**II. Assess for:**
  A. Patterns of sleep/rest

  A. Early detection of problems with sleep/rest leading to complications of fatigue

  B. Verbal/nonverbal clues to sensory deprivation and frustration

  B. Patient may not communicate feelings of frustration in usual manner

**IV. Perform/Provide:**
  A. Diversional activities, talking books, radio, encourage visitors, etc.

  A. ↓ frustration, provides stimulation

**V. Teach patient/family:**
  A. Importance of visitors and conversation and ongoing diversional activities

  A. ↓ frustration, prevents depression associated with sensory deprivation

# ■ Stapedectomy

**DEFINITION:** A surgical procedure to remove a lesion at the footplace of the stapes and implant a prosthesis to replace the portion removed

**CONCEPT/NEED:** Anxiety/Fear

**NURSING DIAGNOSIS:** Anxiety related to loss of hearing

**GOAL:** Reduction in anxiety as evidenced by: verbalization, ability to sleep at night, pulse WNL

| INTERVENTION | RATIONALE |
|---|---|
| **II. Assess for:** | |
| A. Verbal/nonverbal clues to anxiety/fear | A. Patient may be unable to express feelings in the usual manner |
| B. Patient's degree of hearing | B. Necessary for proper condition management |
| C. Patient's level of knowledge about condition/procedure | C. Complete information aids in anxiety reduction |
| D. For presence or degree of vertigo | D. May be present |
| **III. Administer:** | |
| A. Anti-anxiety medication as ordered | A. ↓ anxiety |
| B. Valium IV or Benadryl as ordered | B. Combats vertigo |
| **IV. Perform/Provide:** | |
| A. Listening environment for patient to verbalize feelings | A. ↓ anxiety, promotion of communication |
| B. Comprehensive hearing assessment | B. Determines degree of hearing |
| C. Complete information about condition/procedure | C. ↓ anxiety/fear |
| D. Safety precautions (siderails, obstacles, etc) | D. ↓ potential falls related to vertigo |

## V. Teach patient/family:

A. Vertigo may occur after surgery

A. ↓ anxiety/fear

B. Avoid violent head movements after surgery

B. ↓ vertigo/injury at operative site

C. Hearing will not improve instantly after surgery but in 1–6 weeks

C. ↓ anxiety

D. Avoid flying

D. Sudden pressure changes

E. Not to immerse head in water for 6 weeks (shower also)

E. Infection/re-injury prevention

---

**CONCEPT/NEED:** Safety

**NURSING DIAGNOSIS:** Potential for injury related to vertigo

**GOAL:** Absence of injury as evidenced by: asking for assistance, absence of falls

## INTERVENTION

## RATIONALE

### II. Assess for:

A. Patient's environmental safety (siderails)

A. Prevention of injury related to falls

B. Severity of vertigo

B. May or may not occur

### III. Administer:

A. Antivertigo drugs as ordered

A. Controls vertigo

B. Post-operative position × 24 hours as ordered

B. Promotes drainage, prevents graft displacement

### IV. Perform/Provide:

A. Environment free from obstacles/provide siderails

A. ↑ safety, prevents falls

### V. Teach patient/family:

A. Not to ambulate if having vertigo

A. ↑ safety

B. Not to blow nose, sneeze or violently move head

B. Prevents vertigo, re-injury to surgical site

# ■ Tonsillectomy/Adenoidectomy

**DEFINITION:** The surgical removal of the tonsils and adenoids

**CONCEPT/NEED:** Transport/Circulation

**NURSING DIAGNOSIS:** Alteration in cardiac output related to trauma

**GOAL:** Adequate cardiac output as evidenced by: VS WNL, absence of frank blood

| INTERVENTION | RATIONALE |
|---|---|
| **I. Monitor, describe, record:** | |
| A. TPR (rectal temperature), BP q 2 hr as needed | A. Early detection of hemorrhage and respiratory distress |
| B. Drainage, packing | B. Bright red indicates hemorrhage |
| C. I&O q 4 hr | C. Early detection of hemorrhage and respiratory distress |
| **II. Assess for:** | |
| A. S&S of hemorrhage | A. Early detection, correction of hemorrhage |
| B. S&S of respiratory distress (crowing, retractions, use of respiratory accessory muscle) | B. Early detection and correction of problem |
| C. Condition of tonsillar packing | C. Dislodged or absent |
| D. Aspiration of drainage | D. Detection, prompt correction |
| **III. Administer:** | |
| A. Bedrest as ordered | A. Prevents hemorrhage, packing dislodgement |
| B. Antiemetics as ordered | B. Prevents hemorrhage, packing dislodgement |
| C. NPO for length of time as ordered | C. Prevents hemorrhage, packing dislodgement |
| D. Laxative as ordered | D. Constipation avoidance, possible hemorrhage related to strain |

## IV. Perform/Provide:

A. Inspection of throat with flashlight q 1–2 hr  
A. For bleeding

B. Quiet, restful environment  
B. Prevents excess agitation which could lead to hemorrhage

C. Position as ordered (45 degree head elevation for local anesthetic)  
C. Hemorrhage prevention

## V. Teach patient/family:

A. Not to sneeze, cough or clear throat × 8–10 hours  
A. Prevents packing dislodgement/hemorrhage

B. Expectorate, rather than swallow drainage/phlegm  
B. Prevents aspiration

C. Not to use straw when drinking  
C. Prevents packing dislodgement/hemorrhage

D. Avoid astringent mouth wash  
D. Aids healing

E. Remain in bed 3–4 days after discharge  
E. Prevents hemorrhage

F. Not to smoke  
F. Delays healing vasoconstriction

G. Limit activity  
G. Prevents hemorrhage

H. Avoid constipation  
H. Hemorrhage

I. Stools can appear tarry  
I. From ingested blood

J. S&S of hemorrhage/infection  
J. Early detection and treatment

---

**CONCEPT/NEED:** Pain

**NURSING DIAGNOSIS:** Alteration in comfort: pain related to trauma

**GOAL:** Increased comfort as evidenced by: verbalization, reduced request for pain medication

**INTERVENTION**

**RATIONALE**

## II. Assess for:

A. Characteristics, location and extent of pain  
A. For effective pain management

B. Verbal/nonverbal clues to discomfort  
B. Patient may be unable to express feelings in usual manner

### III. Administer:
A. Analgesics as ordered
B. Ice collar as ordered
C. Diet as ordered, ice chips, water, ice pops, sherbet

A. Pain relief
B. ↓ edema, pain relief
C. Ease of swallowing

### IV. Perform/Provide:
A. Adequate pain assessment
B. Push fluids if possible
C. Position of comfort as permitted

A. Effective pain management
B. Proper hydration/replacement
C. ↑ comfort, pain

### V. Teach patient/family:
A. Large swallows cause less pain than small ones
B. Consume cool liquids until pain subsides
C. Need to progress to soft diet as ordered, as tolerated
D. Good oral hygiene

A. ↓ pain, ↑ comfort

B. ↓ pain, ↑ comfort

C. ↑ comfort

D. ↑ comfort, prevents complications

# INTEGUMENTARY SYSTEM STANDARDS

- Integumentary System Assessment
- Basal Cell/Melanoma
- Decubitus Ulcer
- Dermatitis/Allergic Rash and Eczema/Urticaria/Psoriasis/Acne Vulgaris
- Herpes Simplex/Herpes Zoster
- Skin Infestations/Pediculosis/Scabies/Insect Bites

# ■ Integumentary System Assessment

**DEFINITION:** The collection of a data base concerning the integumentary system and its functional capabilities to be used in identifying nursing problems related to skin integrity and personal hygiene

## INTERVENTION

### I. Interview and investigate for and record past history:
   A. Previous skin conditions such as itching, rashes, tenderness, birthmark changes, warts or moles, athlete's foot, acne
   B. Any hay fever, asthma, allergy, rash or urticaria from foods, medications, insect bites, cosmetics
   C. Tendency for boils, fever blisters
   D. Sensitivity to sun, soaps, deodorants, perfumes
   E. Dryness, oiliness, excessive moisture, body odor, skin color changes
   F. Lumps or growths in the skin, bruising or delayed healing, decreased peripheral circulation
   G. Previous injuries to skin, exposure to chemicals, x-ray treatments
   H. Skin testing and results, responses
   I. Pattern of bathing (tub, shower), frequency, time and kind of soap, tooth paste and shaving cream and/or razor used, lotions and powders used
   J. Medications for skin infections, rashes, lesions (prescribed and OTC)
   K. Previous hair and nail conditions such as alopecia, dandruff, color change, itching, brittleness, ridging, redness, swelling of cuticle
   L. Pattern of hair and nail care, kind of shampoo, rinse, hair set, tint, nail filing and polish, manicures, trimming
   M. Pattern of care of teeth, frequency, times, kind of toothbrush and paste
   N. Family members with skin allergies or diseases, chronic hair, nail, or teeth complaints

### II. Interview and investigate for and record present history:
   A. Chief complaint
   B. Onset and length of illness
   C. Principal signs and symptoms
   D. Knowledge of disease, procedures, and planned therapy
   E. Results of any skin tests, punch biopsies, lesion culture, blood tests
   F. Medications being taken or used for current problem

### III. Inspection for:
    A. Skin color to include cyanosis, jaundice, pallor, pigmentation, redness
    B. Bleeding or bruising, striae, rash, urticaria
    C. Dryness, oiliness, sweating, peeling, scaly
    D. Itching, intactness, cleanliness, odor, exudate, crusting edema, pain, bites
    E. Lesions, lipoma, keloids, warts, moles, boils, blisters, location, grouping, distribution
    F. Nail cleanliness, quantity, texture, thickness, angle, ingrown or hang nails
    G. Hair cleanliness, quantity, texture, distribution, color, baldness, dandruff, odors, brittleness, infestation, lesions, oily, dry

### IV. Palpation for:
    A. Skin temperature of hot, warm, or cold
    B. Texture of skin, rough, bumpy, smooth, thin, thick
    C. Turgor, elasticity, moisture, mobility
    D. Tumors or cysts or any elevations or lumps, skin and scalp
    E. Capillary return in nails
    F. Movement of nail plate when pressed

# ■ Basal Cell/Melanoma

**DEFINITION:** Basal cell is a malignant lesion of the basal cell layer of the epidermis believed to be caused by overexposure to the sun. Melanoma is a malignant tumor of the pigment cells of the skin with a potential for metastasis

**CONCEPT/NEED:** Skin integrity

**NURSING DIAGNOSIS:** Impairment of skin integrity related to destruction of skin layers

**GOAL:** Skin integrity will be maintained as evidenced by: dry crust formation, minimal redness, nonpurulent drainage

| INTERVENTION | RATIONALE |
|---|---|
| II. **Assess for:** | |
| A. Recent change in small papula, mole, or wart | A. Usually crusts and peels |
| B. History of overexposure to sun | B. ↑ risk |
| III. **Administer:** | |
| A. Sunscreen | A. ↓ ultraviolet light absorption |
| B. Antibiotics as ordered | B. ↓ infection after skin surgery |
| IV. **Perform/Provide:** (See Post-Operative Care, p. 17) | |
| V. **Teach patient/family:** | |
| A. Avoid prolonged exposure to sun. When outside, wear protective clothing, e.g., hat, long sleeves. Wear sunscreen when in sun | A. ↓ chance of basal cell disease |
| B. Be alert for changes in moles/warts | B. Potential for basal cell |
| C. Have moles/warts removed | C. Usually where disease begins |

**CONCEPT/NEED:** Anxiety

**NURSING DIAGNOSIS:** Anxiety related to prognosis

**GOAL:** Decreased anxiety as evidenced by: verbalization, pulse WNL, ability to sleep at night

## INTERVENTION

## RATIONALE

II. **Assess for:**
   A. Verbal or nonverbal clues to anxiety
   B. Knowledge of diagnosis, disease process, and treatment

   A. Patient may not be able to openly express feelings
   B. May need more information

IV. **Perform/Provide:**
   A. Listening environment to encourage discussion of feelings
   B. Explanation of proposed treatment

   A. ↓ anxiety

   B. ↓ anxiety

V. **Teach patient/family:**
   A. Importance of follow-up examinations

   A. ↓ chance of early detection

# ■ Decubitus Ulcer

**DEFINITION:** A localized area of the skin, usually at bony prominences, in which epidermal and underlying structures are destroyed because of pressure and immobility

## INTERVENTION

### I. Monitor, describe, record:
A. Condition of skin around ears, heels, back of head, iliac crests, and sacrococcygeal area
B. Fluid and nutritional intake
C. Temperature q 4 hr
D. Daily personal hygiene to include clean, dry skin
E. Changes in WT

### II. Assess for:
A. Amount of activity or movement in bed
B. Deterioration of condition, development of incontinence
C. Obesity or very thin, malnourished
D. Paralysis or state of consciousness
E. Sensory loss, friction
F. Edema
G. Condition of skin, dry, scaly, irritations
H. Position in bed
I. Medications such as sedatives or tranquilizers
J. Symptoms of infection of the skin

### III. Administer:
A. Vitamins and minerals as ordered

### IV. Perform/Provide:
A. Daily skin care per assessment
B. Active and passive exercises
C. Turn, change of position q 2 hr
D. Relief at pressure points such as heel, elbow guards, pillows, pads
E. Preventive devices such as air mattress, sheepskin, fluid-supported mattresses or pads
F. Massage to bony prominences
G. High protein, caloric diet as ordered
H. Lifting instead of sliding or pushing patient

I. Adequate fluid intake according to needs
J. Footboard or bed cradle
K. Clean, dry, and wrinkle-free linens

## V. Teach patient/family:
A. Value of turning and movement
B. Check skin daily for any redness
C. Avoid use of rubbing alcohol, sedatives and tranquilizers, rubber rings or doughnuts
D. Maintain fluid and nutritional intake
E. Keep skin clean, dry and use lotions

# ■ Dermatitis/Allergic Rash and Eczema/Urticaria/Psoriasis/ Acne Vulgaris

**DEFINITION:** Allergy rash and eczema is a condition caused by skin reaction to irritating allergenic materials such as soaps, cosmetics, or ingestion of medications and food causing an allergic reaction. Urticaria is a condition in which wheals (hives) develop as a result of an allergic response to foods or medications. Psoriasis is an inflammatory disease in which production of epidermal cells is accelerated causing a scaling of the skin. Acne vulgaris is a disease of the sebacious glands causing papules, pustules, and lesions on the face, shoulders, and back usually affecting adolescents and young adults

**CONCEPT/NEED:** Infection

**NURSING DIAGNOSIS:** Potential infection related to disturbance of skin layer

**GOAL:** Absence of infection as evidenced by: absence of reddened areas, absence of drainage

| INTERVENTION | RATIONALE |
|---|---|
| II. **Assess for:** | |
| A. Dermatological assessment | A. Identifies possible causes |
| B. General characteristics of lesions, e.g., size, shape, color, number | B. Needed for data base |
| C. Location and distribution of lesions | C. Identifies possible conditions |
| D. Signs of area involved | D. Identifies inflammation from infection |
| E. Extent of area involved | E. The larger the area the more intense the symptoms |
| III. **Administer:** | |
| A. Antihistamines as ordered | A. ↓ itching |

|   |   |
|---|---|
| B. Corticosteroids | B. ↓ inflammations |
| C. Lotions as needed | C. Soothes skin |
| D. Antibiotics as ordered | D. ↓ infection |
| E. Medicated baths | E. Soothes skin |
| F. Ultraviolet treatments | F. ↓ cell replacement process |

**IV. Perform/Provide:**

|   |   |
|---|---|
| A. Safe conditions for baths | A. Insures safety |
| B. Dressings over topical corticosteroids | B. Enhances effectiveness |

**V. Teach patient/family:**

|   |   |
|---|---|
| A. S&S of disease | A. Early detection of disease |
| B. Need to adhere to special diets and treatments | B. Insures patient compliance |
| C. Proper administration of medications as ordered | C. Insures safety |
| D. Proper skin and personal hygiene | D. ↓ chance of infection |

---

**CONCEPT/NEED:** Anxiety
Self-image

**NURSING DIAGNOSIS:** Anxiety related to change in appearance

**GOAL:** Decreased anxiety as evidenced by: verbalization, compliance with treatment, pulse WNL, ability to socialize with peers

| **INTERVENTION** | **RATIONALE** |
|---|---|

**II. Assess for:**

|   |   |
|---|---|
| A. Verbal and nonverbal clues to anxiety, body image | A. Patient may not be able to express feelings openly |
| B. Patient's knowledge about condition, its treatment, and expected outcome | B. ↓ anxiety |

**IV. Provide/Perform:**

|   |   |
|---|---|
| A. Listening environment to encourage patient to verbalize concerns | A. ↓ anxiety |

B. Complete information about patient's condition

B. ↓ anxiety

## V. Teach patient/family:
A. Basic disease process and course of treatment

A. ↓ anxiety and insures patient compliance

# ■ Herpes Simplex/Herpes Zoster

**DEFINITION:** Herpes simplex is a lesion or lesions occurring most frequently on the lips and face and caused by a virus. Another type invades the genitalia. Herpes zoster is an acute painful viral infection of the central nervous system producing vesicular eruptions along a nerve tract

**CONCEPT/NEED:** Pain

**NURSING DIAGNOSIS:** Alteration in comfort: pain related to lesions

**GOAL:** Increased comfort as evidenced by: verbalization, lack of grimacing, decreased request for pain medication

## INTERVENTION

II. **Assess for:**
   A. Burning or itching of infected area
   B. Presence of numerous small vesicles, lesions on lips, nose, vagina, or penis
   C. Development of inflammation and painful vesicles along the course of the posterior root ganglia of selected cranial or spinal nerves
   D. For fever, headache, or malaise

III. **Administer:**
   A. Zovirax (Acyclovir) as ordered
   B. Analgesics
   C. Topical antibiotics
   D. Hourly applications of alcohol
   E. Corticosteroids as ordered

## RATIONALE

A. First signs of herpes

B. Signs of herpes

C. Signs of herpes zoster

D. Serious signs of herpes zoster

A. ↓ duration of outbreak

B. ↓ pain

C. ↓ chance of topical infection

D. Destroys lipoproteins, drying agent

E. ↓ inflammation

## IV. Perform/Provide:
A. Mouthwashes with saline or NaHCO₃ for type I virus

A. Soothes mucous membranes

B. Sitz baths as needed

B. Soothes skin

C. Liquids and soft foods

C. ↓ mouth irritation

D. Bedrest

D. ↓ fatigue

E. Bed cradle as needed

E. ↓ irritation to areas

F. Nonadherent dressings

F. Protects areas from irritation

## V. Teach patient/family:
A. Avoid contact with others during outbreaks of types I and II

A. Sexual contact will spread type II, kissing type I

B. Proper hygiene and not touching lesions

B. Auto-infection will occur

C. Possible complications

C. Pain in orbit is indicative of ophthalmic herpes

# ■ Skin Infestations/Pediculosis/ Scabies/Insect Bites

**DEFINITION:** Pediculosis is the infestation by lice that may appear on three areas of the body—the head (pediculosis capitis), the body (pediculosis corporis), and the pubis (pediculosis pubis). Scabies is the infestation of the skin by the mite. Insect bites include those of bedbugs, fleas, spiders, bees, and other that cause lesions or inflammatory conditions of the skin

**CONCEPT/NEED:** Infection

**NURSING DIAGNOSIS:** Potential infection related to bites

**GOAL:** Absence of infection as evidenced by: lack of redness, scratching

| INTERVENTION | RATIONALE |
|---|---|
| II. Assess for: | |
| A. Excessive scratching by patient | A. Itching is chief symptom |
| B. Part of body involved | B. Patient will need teaching to prevent re-infection |
| C. Presence of very small white nits (eggs) which are attached to hair shafts | C. Indicates lice |
| D. Overcrowded living conditions with poor personal hygiene | D. These organisms thrive in these conditions |
| E. Small, hemorrhagic points on skin | E. Indicative of bites from body lice |
| F. Gray-blue macules 1–3 cm diameter in pubic region | F. Reaction caused by pubic louse |
| G. Crusting, hyperemia, edema, or swollen and tender occipital lymph nodes | G. Secondary infection |
| H. Brownish trails on skin | H. Scabies burrow under skin |
| I. Itching papules in area of skin folds | I. Allergic reaction of scabies |

| | |
|---|---|
| J. Bites, type and number and evidence of stinger | J. Indicates insect bites |
| K. Toxic reactions after bites | K. May indicate allergy |
| L. Vague body pains | L. Indicates tick paralysis |

## III. Administer:

| | |
|---|---|
| A. Gamma-benzene hexachloride topically | A. Destroys lice |
| B. Lotions of menthol and phenol | B. Controls itching |
| C. Topical antibiotics | C. ↓ infection |
| D. Epinephrine for severe allergic reactions | D. For anaphylaxis |

## V. Teach patient/family:

| | |
|---|---|
| A. Proper instructions for cleaning living areas | A. All inhabitants' clothing must be washed. Insecticide must be used |
| B. Proper hygiene | B. ↓ chances of infection |

# ABBREVIATIONS

| | | | |
|---|---|---|---|
| **ABG** | arterial blood gases | **D&C** | dilation and curettage |
| **ACTH** | adrenocorticotropic hormone | **D/C** | discontinue |
| | | **ECG** | electrocardiogram |
| **ADH** | antidiuretic hormone | **EEG** | electroencephalogram |
| **AP** | anteroposterior | **ESR** | erythrocyte sedimentation rate |
| **BID** | 2 times a day | | |
| **BM** | bowel movement | **FF** | force fluids |
| **BMR** | basal metabolic rate | **FROM** | full range of motion |
| **BP** | blood pressure | **GB** | gallbladder |
| **BPH** | benign prostratic hypertrophy | **GI** | gastrointestinal |
| | | **Hct** | hematocrit |
| **bpm** | beats per minute | **Hgb** | hemoglobin |
| **BSP** | bromsuphalein test | **I&O** | intake and output |
| **BUN** | blood urea nitrogen | **ICD** | isocritic dehydrogenase |
| **C&A** | Clinitest and Acetest | **ID** | identification |
| **CAT** | computed axial tomography | **IM** | intramuscular |
| | | **INH** | inhalation |
| **CBC** | complete blood count | **IPPB** | intermittent positive pressure breathing |
| **CHF** | congestive heart failure | | |
| **CHO** | carbohydrate | **IUD** | intrauterine device |
| **CNS** | central nervous system | **IVP** | intravenous pyleogram |
| **COPD** | chronic obstructive pulmonary disease | **kg** | kilogram |
| | | **17-KS** | 17-ketosteroids |
| **CPK** | creatinine phosphokinase | **KUB** | kidney ureter bladder |
| **CV** | cerebrovascular | **L** | liter |
| **CVA** | cerebrovascular accident | **LAP** | leukocyte alkaline phosphatase |
| **CVP** | central venous pressure | | |
| **DB** | deep breathing | **LDH** | lactic dehydrogenase |

| | | | |
|---|---|---|---|
| **LLQ** | left lower quadrant | **RUQ** | right upper quadrant |
| **LMP** | last menstrual period | **S&S** | signs and symptoms |
| **LOC** | level of consciousness | **SGOT** | serum glutamic-oxalo-acetic transaminase |
| **LSD** | lysergic acid diethyla-mide | **SGPT** | serum glutamic-pyruvic transaminase |
| **LUQ** | left upper quadrant | **SL** | sublingual |
| **MI** | myocardial infarction | **SLE** | systemic lupus erythema-tosus |
| **NG** | nasogastric | | |
| **NPO** | nothing by mouth | **SQ** | subcutaneous |
| **O₂** | oxygen | **TB** | tuberculosis |
| **17-OCHS** | 17-hydroxycortico-steroids | **TIBC** | total iron binding capac-ity |
| **OTC** | over the counter | **TID** | 3 times a day |
| **PERL** | pupils equal, react to light | **TOP** | topically |
| | | **TPN** | total parenteral nutrition |
| **PID** | pelvic inflammatory dis-ease | **TPR** | temperature, pulse, res-piration |
| **PMI** | point of maximum inten-sity | **TSH** | thyroid-stimulating hor-mone |
| **PO** | by mouth; orally | **URI** | upper respiratory infec-tion |
| **PPD** | purified protein deriva-tive | **UTI** | urinary tract infection |
| **PRN** | when required | **VD** | venereal disease |
| **PSP** | phenolsulfonphthalein | **VDRL** | venereal disease research laboratory |
| **PT** | prothrombin time | | |
| **PTH** | parathormone | **VS** | vital signs |
| **PTT** | partial thromboplastin time | **WBC** | white blood count |
| | | **WNL** | within normal limits |
| **QD** | every day | **WT** | weight |
| **QID** | 4 times a day | ↓ | decrease; reduce |
| **RBC** | red blood count | ↑ | increase |
| **RLQ** | right lower quadrant | / | per |
| **ROM** | range of motion | | |

# BIBLIOGRAPHY

Bates, B. *A guide to physical examinations* (3rd ed.). Philadelphia: Lippincott, 1983.

Brunner, L. S., & Suddarth, D. S. *Textbook of medical-surgical nursing* (5th ed.). Philadelphia: Lippincott, 1983.

Burns, K. R., & Johnson, P. J. *Health assessment in clinical practice*. Englewood Cliffs, N.J.: Prentice-Hall, 1983.

Carlson, J., et al. *Nursing diagnosis*. Philadelphia: Saunders, 1982.

Carpenito, L. J. *Nursing diagnosis application to clinical practice*. Philadelphia: Lippincott, 1983.

Duke University Hospital Nursing Services. *Guidelines for nursing care: Process and outcome* (2nd ed.). Philadelphia: Lippincott, 1983.

Gordon, M. *Nursing diagnosis process and application*. New York: McGraw-Hill, 1982.

Gordon, M. *Manual of nursing diagnosis 1984–1985*. New York: McGraw-Hill, 1985.

La Monica, E. L. *The humanistic nursing process*. Monterey, Calif.: Wadsworth Health Sciences Division, 1985.

Marriner, A. *The nursing process: A scientific approach to nursing care*. St. Louis: C.V. Mosby, 1983.

Mayers, M. G. *A systematic approach to the nursing care plan* (3rd ed.). Norwalk, Conn.: Appleton-Century-Crofts, 1983.

Mayfield, P. M., & Bond, M. L. *Health assessment, a modular approach*. New York: McGraw-Hill, 1980.

Phipps, W. J., et al. *Medical-surgical nursing concepts and clinical practice*. St. Louis: C. V. Mosby, 1983.

# INDEX